Ultraviolet Radiation in Medicine

Medical Physics Handbooks
Other books in the series

1 **Ultrasonics**
J P Woodcock

2 **Computing Principles and Techniques**
B L Vickery

3 **Physical Principles of Audiology**
P M Haughton

4 **Urodynamics**
D J Griffiths

5 **Thermoluminescence Dosimetry**
A F McKinlay

6 **Fundamentals of Radiation Dosimetry**
J R Greening

7 **Radiotherapy Treatment Planning**
R F Mould

8 **Nuclear Particles in Cancer Treatment**
J F Fowler

9 **Physics of the Circulation**
J O Rowan

10 **The Evaluation of Medical Images**
A Ll Evans

Series Editor: **Professor J M A Lenihan**
Department of Clinical Physics and Bio-Engineering
West of Scotland Health Boards, Glasgow

Medical Physics Handbooks 11

Ultraviolet Radiation in Medicine

B L Diffey
Dryburn Hospital, Durham

Adam Hilger Ltd, Bristol
in collaboration with the
Hospital Physicists' Association

British Library Cataloguing in Publication Data

Diffey, B L
Ultraviolet radiation in medicine.—
(Medical physics handbooks; 11 ISSN 0143-0203)
1. Ultra-violet rays—Physiological effect
2. Ultra-violet rays—Therapeutic use
3. Phototherapy
I. Title II. Series
612′.01448 R895,A5

ISBN 0-85274-535-4

Published by Adam Hilger Ltd,
Techno House, Redcliffe Way, Bristol BS1 6NX

The Adam Hilger book-publishing imprint is owned by
The Institute of Physics

Printed in Great Britain by
Page Bros (Norwich) Ltd

Contents

Preface

The aims of this book are to indicate those areas in which ultraviolet radiation is used in medicine together with the physical principles governing its production, application and measurement. The book is intended primarily as an introduction to the subject for medical physicists, but it is hoped that some of the material will be of interest to dermatologists, physiotherapists, photobiologists, biophysicists and to some workers in the cosmetic industry.

The first chapter is a brief historical survey of some of the important developments in phototherapy, photophysics, photochemistry and photobiology, particularly within the past 100 years or so.

The factors affecting the quality and quantity of natural ultraviolet radiation are covered in Chapter 2, together with the physics associated with the production of artificial ultraviolet radiation. Chapter 3 is concerned with the properties of various optical components that may be used in medical ultraviolet photobiology. The second half of this chapter is devoted to the clinical irradiation monochromator, a tool which is being used increasingly in photodermatological investigations. Ultraviolet radiation dosimetry is discussed in Chapter 4. The physical principles governing the action of ultraviolet radiation detectors are described, followed by an examination of spectral irradiance and biologically-weighted irradiance measurement techniques.

The observable biological effects of external ultraviolet radiation exposure in man are described in Chapter 5. These effects are limited to the skin and to the eyes and this chapter outlines the optical properties and the recognisable short-term and long-term effects of UV exposure of these organs. Ultraviolet radiation is employed in a variety of situations in medicine under headings which can be classified broadly as therapy, diagnosis and non-clinical applications. Some of these currently-used applications are discussed in Chapter 6. Finally, Chapter 7 reports on some recent studies of personal exposure to environmental ultraviolet radiation and the current safety standards associated with occupational exposure to ultraviolet radiation.

The intention of the book is to emphasize the practical nature of the subject and to this end liberal use has been made of diagrams and photographs where it was felt that these would be helpful to the reader.

B L Diffey

Acknowledgments

Since my interest in ultraviolet radiation physics and biology first began some eight years ago, I have been extremely fortunate in the help and co-operation that I have received from many scientists, clinicians and industrialists.

It is always difficult to select individuals for special thanks but I am especially indebted to Mr J R Corfield who first encouraged my interest in the subject and in whose Medical Physics Department at the Kent and Canterbury Hospital much of my work was carried out. Likewise I am grateful to Professor K Boddy who continues to support my efforts in this area.

I should like to thank, in particular, Dr A Davis and Professor I A Magnus for many years of fruitful collaboration in the field of ultraviolet radiation measurement. Professor Magnus also deserves my thanks for reading the manuscript of this book.

Finally I should like to record my appreciation to Mrs S Lumsdon for carefully typing the manuscript, and to my wife June for her encouragement during the preparation of this book.

1 Ultraviolet Radiation in Medicine: Historical Introduction

In 1666 Isaac Newton '. . . procured me a Triangular glass-Prisme, to try therewith the celebrated Phaenomena of Colours' and opened up a new era into the scientific investigation of light. It was not until 1801 that Johann Ritter discovered the ultraviolet region of the solar spectrum by showing that chemical action was caused by some form of energy in the dark portion beyond the violet. It had been in the previous year, 1800, that Sir William Herschel had demonstrated the existence of radiation beyond the red end of the visible spectrum, a component now known as infrared radiation.

1.1 The Ultraviolet Spectrum

Ultraviolet radiation (UVR) is part of the electromagnetic spectrum and lies between the visible and the x-ray regions. Different wavebands in the ultraviolet spectrum show enormous variations in causing biological damage and for this reason the UV spectrum is divided into three spectral regions; UV-A, UV-B and UV-C.

The notion to divide the ultraviolet spectrum into different spectral regions was first put forward at the Copenhagen meeting of the Second International Congress on Light held during August 1932 (Coblentz 1932). It was recommended that three spectral regions be defined as follows:

UV-A	400–315 nm
UV-B	315–280 nm
UV-C	<280 nm

Various regulatory authorities including the International Commission on Illumination (CIE), the National Institute for Occupational Safety and Health (NIOSH) in the United States, and the Health and Safety Executive (HSE) and the National Radiological Protection Board (NRPB) in the United Kingdom, have endorsed these regions, with the slight modification that the lower limit of the UV-C region is taken to be 100 nm by the CIE, HSE and NRPB, and 200 nm by the NIOSH. Radiation in the spectral region 100–200 nm (the vacuum UV) is readily attenuated in air with little opportunity to produce direct biological effects, and so the lower limit of the UV-C region for practical purposes is not critical.

The development of environmental photobiology has prompted some workers (Parrish *et al* 1978) to redefine the boundaries of the three spectral regions as follows:

UV-A	400–320 nm
UV-B	320–290 nm
UV-C	290–200 nm

The upper limit of the UV-B region has been extended to 320 nm, since most acute and chronic effects of sunlight exposure on biological systems are believed to occur at wavelengths less than 320 nm, whilst the division between the UV-B and UV-C regions has been set at 290 nm since this wavelength is the approximate lower limit of terrestrial radiation. Yet another publication (WHO 1979) has defined the UV-B region as 280–320 nm. Although the divisions between the spectral regions are not necessarily rigid it would seem sensible to adopt international recommendations and so the convention in this book is to follow the British authorities, viz:

Spectral region	Also known as	Range of wavelengths (nm)
UV-A	longwave or 'blacklight'	400–315
UV-B	middlewave or 'erythemal'	315–280
UV-C	shortwave or 'germicidal'	280–100

1.2 Ancient Concepts of Sunlight and Health

The worship of the sun as a health-bringing deity is probably as old as man himself. Almost all early peoples revered the sun, especially in the cradle of civilization around the Mediterranean basin, where the sun shines with a dependable regularity. In fact, the word 'radiation' stems from Aton Ra, the Egyptian sun god established during the Fifth Dynasty (2750 BC). And from Helios, the Greek god of light and sun, is derived the word 'heliotherapy' which means healing by exposure to the sun's rays.

Possibly the earliest medical association with sunlight is the observation of Herodotus, who, in 525 BC, related the strength of the skull to sunlight exposure. Sunbathing was prescribed by many early physicians for such diverse conditions as epilepsy, jaundice and obesity. During the eighteenth and nineteenth centuries the therapeutic benefits of sunlight exposure were beginning to be understood on a scientific basis, particularly in the treatment of rickets. However it was not until the end of the nineteenth century that the importance of the ultraviolet component of sunlight was realised. This discovery was made by the Danish physician Niels Finsen (1860–1904) whom many regard as the father of modern ultraviolet therapy.

1.3 Early Phototherapy

The foundations of modern-day ultraviolet phototherapy began with the work of Niels Finsen (*see* figure 1.1) who completed his first article about light, *On the Influence of the Light on the Skin*, in the spring of 1893. In a series of articles published between 1893–96 Finsen stressed that it was the ultraviolet radiation in the solar spectrum that was responsible for sunburn and not the radiant heat, as the name implies. In parallel with his scientific investigations Finsen was also an active clinician. He is best remembered for his successful treatment of lupus vulgaris (tuberculosis of the skin, mainly on the face) and in 1903 was awarded the Nobel Prize for Medicine in recognition of this work. The photograph shown in figure 1.2 was taken about 1895 and shows patients with lupus vulgaris under Finsen's care being treated with sunlight. Finsen realised that the ultraviolet component of sunlight was variable and so turned his attention to the carbon arc lamp as a source of artificial UVR. Figure 1.3 shows a patient with lupus vulgaris undergoing actinotherapy (treatment with artificial sources of radiation) with one of these early 'Finsen lamps'. At the centre of the assembly is a carbon arc lamp. Radiating out from the lamp are several tubes incorporating quartz lenses which contain solutions of copper sulphate or methylene blue.

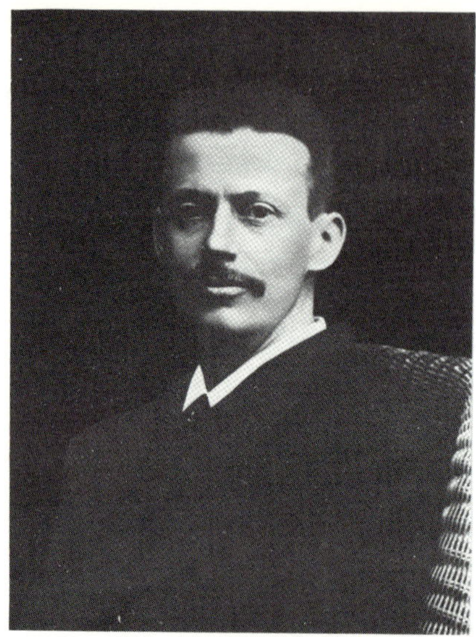

Figure 1.1 Niels Ryberg Finsen, 1860–1904. (Courtesy of the Finsen Institute, Copenhagen, Denmark.)

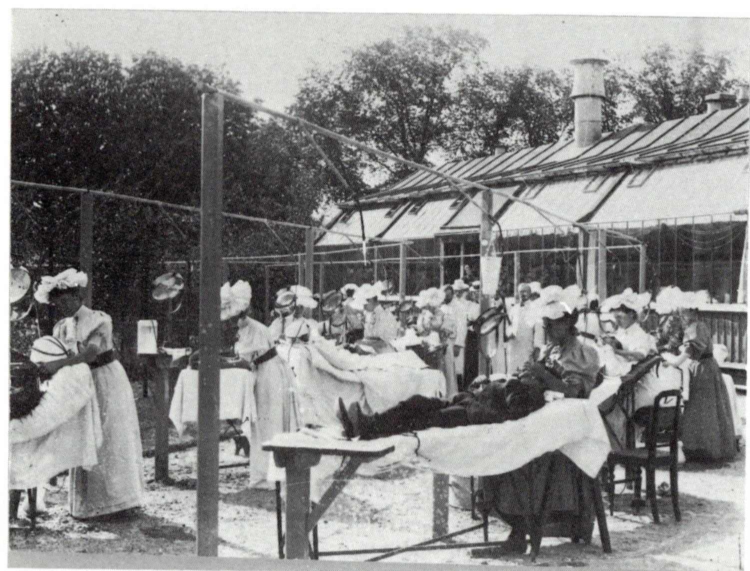

Figure 1.2 Treatment of lupus vulgaris with sunlight, *c* 1895. (Courtesy of the Finsen Institute, Copenhagen, Denmark.)

These solutions act to absorb the infrared radition and so maximise the ultraviolet radiation while preventing a thermal burn. Finsen also used a quartz lens to apply pressure in order to remove the blood from the skin and so to increase penetration of the ultraviolet radiation.

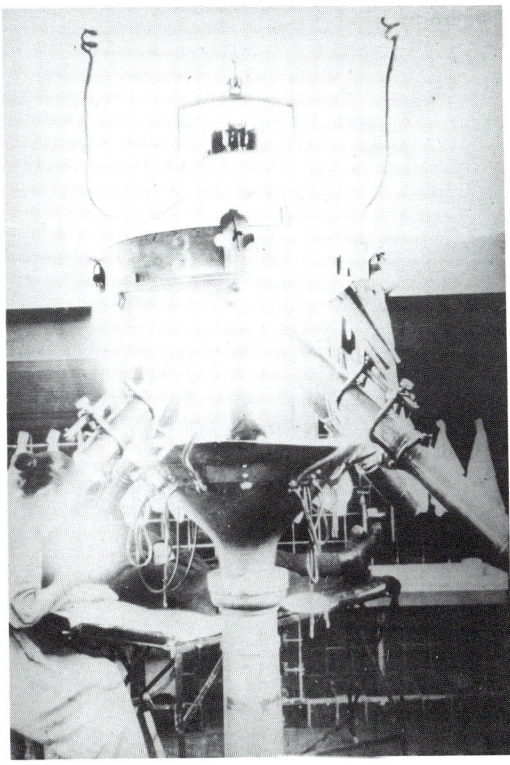

Figure 1.3 The carbon arc developed by Niels Finsen being used for actinotherapy. (Courtesy of the Finsen Institute, Copenhagen, Denmark.)

As well as being a skillful clinician, Finsen made several fundamental contributions to the physics of phototherapy. For example, he showed that, instead of using ordinary carbon electrodes in the lamp, it was possible to bore out the carbon sticks and fill them with burned lime, thereby increasing the intensity of the UVR.

Regrettably, Finsen suffered poor health for most of his life and was too ill to receive his Nobel Prize at the annual festival, but instead had it presented by the Swedish–Norwegian consul on his 43rd birthday, December 15, 1903. Less than a year later he died.

Following the pioneering work of Finsen, the early part of the twentieth century saw the rapid expansion of heliotherapy and actinotherapy throughout Europe and the United States of America. In his book on sunlight and health published in 1926, Saleeby discusses with much enthusiasm the benefits of heliotherapy and in particular describes the work of Dr Rollier at Leysin in the Alpes Vaudoises, whose experience in twenty years of successful treatment of surgical turberculosis by natural sunlight has included '. . . many extreme cases of spinal tuberculosis, with paralysed lower limbs, tuberculosis of every other part of the body, of course, including the lungs, rickets, many skin diseases, varicose ulcers of the longest standing, wounds of war, non-healing operative wounds, osteomyelitis, bed-sores and so on'(Saleeby 1926). In the preface to the third edition of his book Saleeby notes the formation of the Sunlight League in London in 1924 and states as one of its aims 'the education of the public to the appreciation of sunlight as a means of health; teaching the nation that sunlight is Nature's universal disinfectant, as well as a stimulant and tonic'.

The practice of actinotherapy continued to expand through the middle part of the twentieth century and was accompanied by an enormous literature on the subject during the 1920s and 1930s. This rapid growth is reflected by the many revisions of the handbook *Actinotherapy Technique* first published by the Sollux Publishing Company in 1933 and reprinted for the ninth time (7th edition) in 1949. Most of the irradiation protocols for the countless number of diseases described in this book are now of historical interest only. The advent of effective antibiotics and the realisation that the successes claimed in many of these diseases were little more than anecdotal have resulted today in a much reduced role of ultraviolet radiation in clinical medicine. On the other hand one of the major contributions to dermatological practice for many years has been the recent introducton of a treatment for the common skin disease psoriasis, known as photochemotherapy; the combination of ultraviolet radiation and photoactive drugs producing a beneficial effect in the skin.

1.4 Early Photophysics

One of the reasons for the widespread use of actinotherapy in medicine was the availability of artificial sources of ultraviolet radiation. The first arc was demonstrated in the early part of the nineteenth century by Humphrey Davy, who created an electrical discharge in air between charcoal electrodes. In 1835 Wheatstone observed the intense light which is emitted when mercury is vapourised in the electric arc. A mercury lamp incorporating carbon electrodes was patented by E H Jackson of Soho in 1852. In the following year Christopher Binks patented a lamp which was similar, but contained mercury electrodes. Several advances were made in lamp technology around the turn of the century, including the development by W C Heraeus who, in 1903, devised an improved way to fuse quartz. This allowed E L Kromayer to evaluate the therapeutic performance of the quartz mercury vapour lamp, which led to his design in 1905 of the water-cooled lamp which still bears his name. The first fluorescent lamps did not appear until the late 1930s, but their development was inhibited by the advent of the second world war. Consequently ultraviolet fluorescent lamps did not find a place in phototherapy until the 1950s.

Early radiation dosimetry in phototherapy was accomplished by noting the ability of a source of radiation to produce an erythema (sunburn) in human skin. In fact this method is still used in most physiotherapy departments at the start of a course of UV treatment on an individual. This 'unit' is subject to a large uncertainty in accuracy since there are great variations in photosensitivity from one person to another, and the biological effects of ultraviolet radiation vary enormously with changes in the wavelength of the radiation. As a result the Council of Physical Therapy of the American Medical Association introduced in the 1930s the 'Erythemal Unit' (EU), which was defined as 10 μW of monochromatic radiation of wavelength 296.7 nm (a characteristic line in the mercury vapour spectrum effective in producing erythema). The Illumination Engineering Society and the International Commission on Illumination adopted the term E-viton for this quantity of radiant flux, and so 1 E-viton is the radiant flux which produces the same erythemal effect as 10 μW of 296.7 nm radiation. The E-viton was a biological unit in that it represented the integrated spectral radiant flux of a source weighted by the ability of the component wavelengths to produce an erythema. The radiant exposure, or dose, of ultraviolet radiation is the product of E-vitons with time. One EU per cm^2 or 1 E-viton per cm^2 were adopted as the unit of erythemal flux intensity and termed the 'Finsen'. It requires about 15,000 $\mu W\,s\,cm^{-2}$ of radiation of wavelength 296.7 nm to produce a just perceptible erythema on untanned Caucasian skin; this is equivalent to 1500 E-viton s cm^{-2} or 1500 Finsen s. Modern UVR dosimetry uses the terminology of radiometry and the SI system of units (*see* Chapter 4). Hence this radiant exposure is now expressed as 150 J m^{-2}.

1.5 Early Photochemistry

The production of a biological effect following ultraviolet irradiation involves an intermediate stage whereby the molecules in the system absorb the radiation which often initiates a host of chemical reactions. Over the past 200 years various laws have been postulated which have played an important role in the development of photochemical concepts.

In 1818 Grotthus formulated the so-called first law of photochemistry, which is that only the radiations which are absorbed are effective in promoting a photochemical change. This relationship was experimentally verified by Draper in 1839 and so is sometimes referred to as the Grotthus–Draper law. The second law of photochemistry, or Bunsen–Roscoe reciprocity law, followed shortly afterwards and states that when the product of the intensity and the exposure time is constant, the photochemical effect is the same. Perhaps it is worth noting here that this law does not hold for erythema resulting from sunlight exposure (Magnus 1976) but has been shown to hold over a factor of 10^7 in intensity for erythema produced by artificial radiation in mouse skin (Claesson *et al* 1958).

The Lambert–Beer law of absorption, published in the mid-nineteenth century, states that the fraction of incident radiation which is absorbed by a substance in solution is independent of the radiation intensity and increases proportionally with increase in concentration of the substance.

The quantum law, familiar to all physicists, was formulated by the German physicist Max Planck in 1901 and states that radiation is emitted in discrete bundles, or quanta, of energy. This law laid the foundations for Stark in 1908 and Einstein in 1912 to postulate the law of photochemical equivalence, which states that each quantum of radiation absorbed by a molecule activates one molecule in the primary step of a photochemical process. It should be stressed that an activated molecule does not necessarily undergo a chemcial reaction; on the other hand one activated molecule may cause the reaction of many other molecules. The number of molecules of reactant consumed or product formed per quantum of radiation absorbed is expressed by the quantum yield.

Finally the technique of flash photolysis developed by Porter and Norrish in 1949 has enabled short-lived ($<10^{-9}$ s) photochemical intermediates to be identified.

1.6 Early Photobiology

Photobiology is the study of the effect of non-ionising radiation, chiefly the ultraviolet and visible regions, on living systems. The subject is vast, covering biological disciplines from botany, through zoology, to medicine. This section will limit itself to a discussion of some of the more important developments in medical photobiology.

The first report of the bactericidal effect of sunlight was made by Downes and Blunt in 1877. They were not able to determine whether it was the light or heat that was effective. This was demonstrated by Duclaux in 1885 and, to a greater extent, by Ward in 1892, who showed that the most efficient bactericidal action occurred in the ultraviolet. Finsen employed the bactericidal effect of UVR as a biological dosimetry system in his study of the UV transmission properties of quartz and window glass. By this means he was able to demonstrate that the radiation from a carbon arc, whether unfiltered or passed through quartz, exhibited similar bactericidal effects, whereas almost no effect was observed on the bacteria exposed to radiation through the window glass. Two of Finsen's co-workers, Valdemar Bie and Sophus Bang, continued these studies and established that UVR of wavelengths less than 300 nm, especially around 250 nm, were most effective in killing bacteria. It wasn't until 1929 that Gates published an action spectrum for the bactericidal effect of ultraviolet radiation and confirmed the earlier observations of Bie and Bang.

Probably the best known effect of ultraviolet radiation on man is the production of erythema, or sunburn. In 1859 Charcot suggested that erythema was produced by the chemical rays of an electric arc, although his hypothesis was not proven for almost 20 years. Again, the pioneering work of Finsen showed that natural sunburn was only produced by the ultraviolet component of sunlight. The erythema action spectrum in human skin, that is the relative effectiveness of different wavelengths in producing sunburn, was first determined by the German physicist Karl Hausser and his colleague Wilhelm Vahle in 1921. They were the first to employ an irradiation monochromator for action spectra studies and used a mercury lamp as the light source in conjunction with a double quartz prism monochromator. A photograph of their monochromator is shown in figure 1.4 and on the right hand side of this photograph can be seen the clamp where the subject's arm was kept still during the long exposures that were necessary! Their results showed that the UV-A and visible spectra were ineffective in producing erythema and that there was a rapid increase in skin sensitivity as the radiation wavelength approached 300 nm, with a maximal sensitivity at 297 nm. The sensitivity dropped sharply again at wavelengths below 297 nm, reaching a minimum at 280 nm but thereafter increasing slowly to reach a second, but lesser, peak at 254 nm. In addition to their work on the erythema action spectrum, Hausser and Vahle also studied the main features of the dose-response curve and the time course of erythema, together with measurements on the action spectrum for melanogenesis (suntan). There followed a spate of publications in the 1920s and 1930s on the erythema action spectrum, all showing much the same curve as Hausser and Vahle. More recent investigations in the 1960s and 1970s have confirmed the long wavelength cut-off at around 310 nm but have found wavelengths around 250 nm to be more effective than those around 297 nm (*see* Chapter 5).

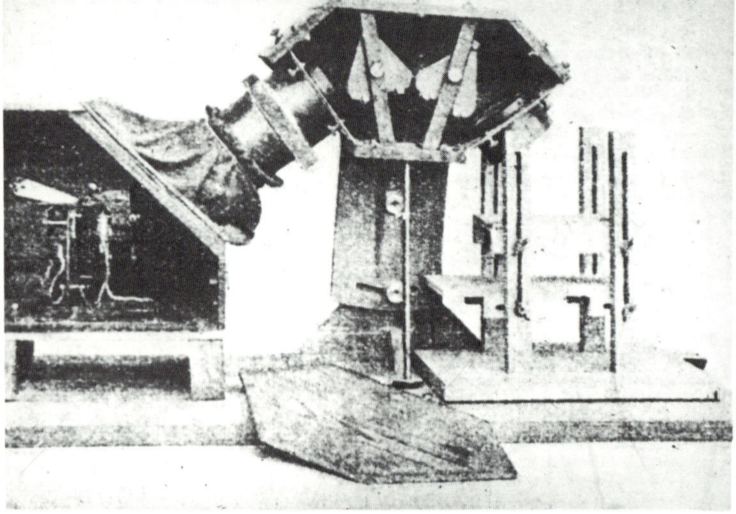

Figure 1.4 The monochromator used by Hausser and Vahle in the determination of the erythema action spectrum in human skin in 1921 (from Hausser and Vahle 1922.)

Perhaps the most insidious effect of ultraviolet radiation on man is the induction of skin cancer. The dermatologist Unna was the first to recognise the relationship between precancerous development of the skin and sunlight exposure in 1894. Much of the knowledge that we have on the mechanism of ultraviolet radiation induced cancers of the skin results from the the notable work of the physiologist Harold Blum in the 1940s and 1950s. Blum carried out several careful investigations into the UV dose-response relationship of skin tumours in mice. He also established that it is those wavelengths shorter than 320 nm which are effective in producing skin cancer; this is perhaps not surprising when it is realised that many important compounds, notably the nucleic acids and proteins, strongly absorb these wavelengths.

2 The Production of Ultraviolet Radiation

Ultraviolet radiation (UVR) may be produced either by the heating of a body to an incandescent temperature or by the excitation of a gas discharge. Recently lasers have been developed which emit intense, coherent beams of monochromatic UVR, although the availability and prohibitive cost of these devices has limited their use to research applications. This chapter will cover the production of incoherent (non-laser) UVR and will begin with the most common source of ultraviolet exposure to man—sunlight.

2.1 Solar Radiation

The radiant energy received from the sun is responsible for the development and continued existence of life on earth. The spectral distribution as well as the total amount of energy reaching the Earth's surface are both important factors in our environment.

The intensity of the solar radiation on a surface normal to the Sun's direction, outside the Earth's atmosphere and at the Earth's mean distance from the Sun is called the solar constant. Recent determinations of the solar constant have yielded a value of $1.351 \pm 0.028\ \mathrm{kW\,m^{-2}}$. About two-thirds of this energy actually reaches the surface of the Earth, the remainder being reflected, scattered or absorbed in the atmosphere. Of this energy about 50% lies in the visible spectrum and about 5% is in the ultraviolet. At noon during the summer in the UK, the irradiance on an unshaded horizontal surface is around $40\ \mathrm{W\,m^{-2}}$ in the UV-A and less than $2\ \mathrm{W\,m^{-2}}$ in the UV-B.

The solar radiation which reaches the surface of the Earth consists of a direct component (sunlight) and a diffuse, or scattered, component (skylight). The total radiation, sunlight plus skylight, is designated global radiation.

The global ultraviolet radiation is attenuated in the atmosphere principally by the following effects:

(a) absorption by atmospheric ozone which is concentrated in a layer between 10 and 50 km above sea level with a concentration maximum of about 10 ppm at an altitude of about 25 km. The total amount of atmospheric ozone is variable but generally equivalent to a layer about 0.3 cm thick at standard temperature and pressure (STP). The absorption of UVR by ozone is important for wavelengths less than 330 nm, where the values of the ozone absorption coefficient increase rapidly with decreasing wavelength so that there is practically no radiation with wavelengths less than 295 nm which reaches the Earth's surface;

(b) Rayleigh scattering caused by oxygen, nitrogen and other molecular components of the atmosphere, where the scattering particle is small compared with the wavelength of the radiation;

(c) Mie scattering caused by dust, aerosols, water droplets and other particles of diameter comparable to the wavelength of the radiation.

In addition to the above effects, the degree of cloud cover and ground reflection will also affect the diffuse component of the global radiation.

2.1.1 Variation in solar UVR

The approximate spectral irradiance of global radiation at sea level for the Sun directly overhead (solar zenith angle of zero degrees) is shown in figure 2.1. However the ultraviolet component of global radiation, particularly in the UV-B region, is subject to considerable variation in both spectral content and irradiance. Some of the factors which influence these variations will now be dicussed.

2.1.1.1 Geometrical and astronomical variations. The intensity of solar UVR outside the atmosphere will be dependent on the distance from the Sun to the Earth. This distance shows annual variations of ±3.5% and depends only on the day of the year. Extraterrestrial solar intensity is highest on January 1st corresponding to the smallest Sun-to-Earth separation (perihelion) and lowest on or about July 3rd when the separation is a maximum (aphelion). Clearly then, it is apparent to those of us residing in the Northern Hemisphere that this factor has negligible influence on the intensity of solar UVR which actually reaches the Earth's surface. Also, variations in the Sun itself, estimated at ±1.5% overall, have a similar negligible effect.

2.1.1.2 Attenuation by the atmosphere. If the diffuse component is neglected, then the spectral irradiance $I(\lambda)$ of solar radiation which reaches the Earth can be represented approximately as

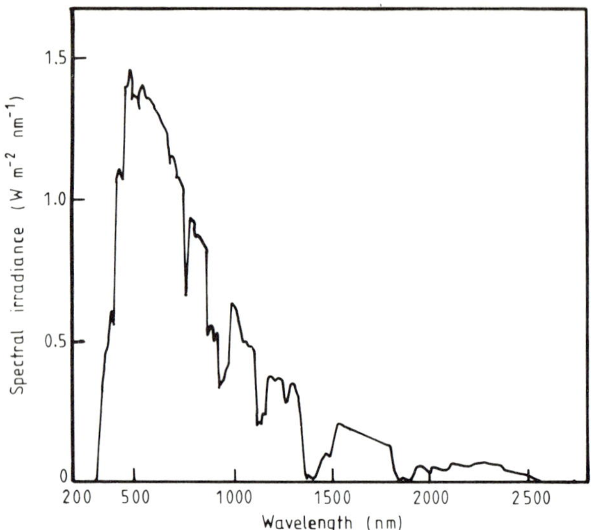

Figure 2.1 The spectral irradiance of global radiation at the Earth's surface for the sun directly overhead (optical air mass equal to 1.0.)

$$I(\lambda) = I_0(\lambda) \cos\theta \exp\{-[({}_\lambda\tau_R + {}_\lambda\tau_m)\, dm_\theta + {}_\lambda\tau_o X m_\theta]\}, \qquad (2.1)$$

where $I_0(\lambda)$ is the spectral irradiance of extraterrestrial radiation at wavelength λ; θ is the solar zenith angle, i.e. the angle between the Sun's rays and the normal to the Earth (the solar zenith angle = 90°—solar altitude); ${}_\lambda\tau_R$, ${}_\lambda\tau_m$ and ${}_\lambda\tau_o$ are the extinction coefficients at wavelength λ for Rayleigh scattering, Mie scattering and ozone absorption respectively; d is the thickness of the atmosphere normal to the Earth; X is the thickness of the ozone layer at STP; and m_θ is the relative optical air mass given approximately as

$$m_\theta = \sec\theta. \qquad (2.2)$$

With the Sun directly overhead the air mass is equal to 1, but at dawn or dusk, with a solar zenith angle of say, 60°, the air mass is equal to 2; that is, the Sun's rays have then twice the thickness of atmosphere to traverse.

For wavelengths below about 330 nm attenuation by ozone assumes much greater significance than either Rayleigh or Mie scattering, and increases rapidly with decreasing wavelength. The solar spectral irradiance for these wavelengths decreases more rapidly as the solar zenith angle, θ, increases, and so the intensity of wavelengths in the UV-B are much more strongly dependent on the height of the sun in the sky than are UV-A or visible wavelengths. This is why the sunburning effectiveness of sunlight, due primarily to UV-B (*see* Chapter 5), is about 100 times more intense in the summer, when the sun is higher in the sky than in the winter.

2.1.1.3 Scattering in the atmosphere. The calculation of the scattered radiation which reaches the Earth's surface is mathematically very difficult, due to multiple Rayleigh and Mie scattering in the atmosphere. Both effects are wavelength dependent and indeed, it is the λ^{-4} dependence of Rayleigh scatttering which results in a blue sky on a clear day.

The relative contributions of the scattered and direct components to the total global radiation are shown in figure 2.2 for UV-B and UV-A. It can be seen that at noon in the summer in the UK (solar altitude approximately equal to 60°) the direct and scattered components are

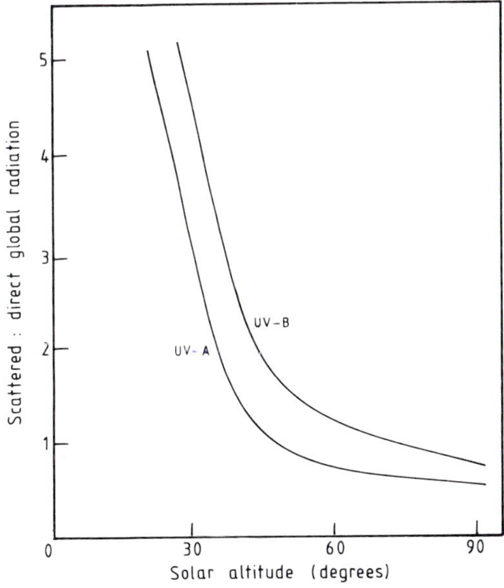

Figure 2.2 The ratio of scattered to direct global UV-A and UV-B on a horizontal surface at sea level as a function of solar altitude (ozone layer thickness equivalent to 0.32 cm at STP.)

approximately equal, but that in the early morning and late afternoon (solar altitude ~25°) the scattered component is significantly larger than the direct component, particularly for the UV-B. In fact, the importance of the scattered UV-B component is a reason why it may be possible to become sunburnt while in the shade in an area to which a large region of the sky is exposed.

2.1.1.4 Clouds. The presence of clouds in the sky can result in a reduced UV irradiance, although the relative changes in the UV region are not very great as far the total irradiance is concerned, since the water content of clouds will attenuate the infrared component of sunlight much more effectively than the UV component. The risk of overexposure may be increased under these conditions because the sensation of heat that acts as a warning will be diminished.

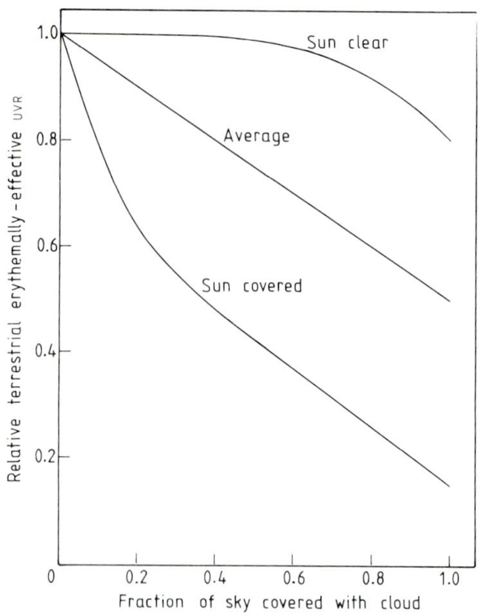

Figure 2.3 The relative amounts of erythemally-effective UVR reaching sea level as a function of the fraction of the sky covered with cloud. The central, sloping curve is an average estimate for the UK, while the upper and lower curves show the approximate range of instantaneous values as a cloud covers or exposes the sun.

Even with heavy cloud cover the scattered UV penetration is seldom less than 10% of that under a clear sky and light clouds scattered over a blue sky make little difference to the sunburning (erythemal) effectiveness of sunlight unless a cloud covers the sun. If the sun is covered by a cloud the direct solar radiation will be widely scattered but the total erythemal sky radiation will still be about 50% of the global radiation on a clear day.

The effect of cloud cover can be summarised in figure 2.3, which shows the relative amounts of erythemally-effective UVR (i.e. UV-B radiation) reaching sea-level as a function of the fraction of sky covered with cloud. The central, sloping straight line is an average estimate for the UK, while the upper and lower lines show the approximate range of instantaneous values as a cloud covers or exposes the sun.

2.1.1.5 Surface reflection. Fresh snow on the ground can act as an efficient reflector of both UV-A and UV-B and may scatter in excess of 80% of the incident radiation upwards, which can lead to severe burning.

A green grass lawn scatters about 3% of the incident UV radiation. Sand is about 25% as reflective as the sky and so sitting under an umbrella on the beach can lead to sunburn from both scattered UV-B from the sky and reflected UV-B from the sand.

Contrary to popular belief, water will reflect no more than 5% of the incident erythemal UVR. However at least 40% is transmitted through 50 cm of clear water, as many bathers at the seaside have experienced to their discomfort.

2.1.1.6 Altitude. In general each 300 m increase in altitude will increase the erythemal effectiveness of global UVR by about 4%. At an altitude of 1500 m therefore the global UV-B is around 20% greater than it is at sea-level. In fact it is the intensity of the direct component which increases with altitude as the scattered component decreases by about 1% per 300 m.

2.1.2 Calculation of the global UV environment

An appreciation of the spectral distribution of global UVR for a variety of spatial and temporal situations is important in the clinical management of sunlight-provoked lesions which may be either idiopathic or drug-induced. It is evident from the previous section that a rigorous theoretical determination of the global UV spectrum is extremely complex, although computer models of the UV environment have been described by several workers (McCullough 1970; Green *et al* 1974; Green *et al* 1980).

In this section a set of empirical equations are presented which are based upon the most extensive set of measurements of global UV spectral irradiance yet available (Bener 1972). The equations will enable approximate values of the spectral distribution of natural UVR to be calculated for any time of day, day of year and geographical latitude. The limitation of the equations is that they apply to clear-day conditions (i.e. no cloud cover) encountered at sea-level and for no reflection from the ground. Nevertheless they are readily implemented on a digital computer and are certainly adequate for assessing the relative importance of solar radiation in initiating a given photobiological response in a variety of situations.

2.1.2.1 Development of the equations. The spectral distribution of ultraviolet global radiation (in $W\,m^{-2}\,nm^{-1}$) on a horizontal surface at wavelength λ, solar altitude h and total amount of atmospheric ozone χ, is denoted by $G(\lambda, h, \chi)$. Values of this function for 0.32 cm ozone at selected wavelengths and solar altitudes are given in table 2.1, and are reproduced from the measured data of Bener.

Table 2.1 Approximate values of the spectral distribution of global ultraviolet radiation (in $W\,m^{-2}\,nm^{-1}$) for a cloudless sky at sea level and a total amount of atmospheric ozone of 0.32 cm at STP (after Bener 1972).

Wavelength (nm)	Solar altitude 5°	10°	20°	40°	60°	90°
297.5	0.000	0.000	0.000	0.116(−3)	0.107(−2)	0.218(−2)
300.0	0.000	0.000	0.255(−4)	0.766(−3)	0.404(−2)	0.720(−2)
302.5	0.715(−5)	0.183(−4)	0.116(−3)	0.363(−2)	0.129(−1)	0.208(−1)
305.0	0.253(−4)	0.794(−4)	0.661(−3)	0.117(−1)	0.343(−1)	0.497(−1)
307.5	0.934(−4)	0.293(−3)	0.220(−2)	0.248(−1)	0.604(−1)	0.822(−1)
310.0	0.208(−3)	0.706(−3)	0.523(−2)	0.399(−1)	0.966(−1)	0.130
312.5	0.613(−3)	0.242(−2)	0.136(−1)	0.746(−1)	0.146	0.186
315.0	0.131(−2)	0.492(−2)	0.251(−1)	0.102	0.189	0.241
317.5	0.267(−2)	0.101(−1)	0.365(−1)	0.132	0.237	0.293
320.0	0.449(−2)	0.144(−1)	0.506(−1)	0.166	0.277	0.339
325.0	0.103(−1	0.271(−1)	0.771(−1)	0.220	0.379	0.465
330.0	0.192(−1)	0.462(−1)	0.115	0.281	0.441	0.535
340.0	0.232(−1)	0.532(−1)	0.125	0.309	0.475	0.578
360.0	0.303(−1)	0.634(−1)	0.135	0.331	0.515	0.624
380.0	0.335(−1)	0.665(−1)	0.142	0.374	0.600	0.727

Note. (−5) means $\times 10^{-5}$

An estimate of UV spectral irradiance for any other thickness of ozone and solar altitude may be expressed as

$$G(\lambda, h, \chi) = A(\lambda, h)F(\lambda, h, \chi) \tag{2.3}$$

where $A(\lambda, h)$ is a logarithmic interpolation function between the tabulated values of spectral intensity at wavelength λ and 0.32 cm ozone for any solar altitude h, and $F(\lambda, h, \chi)$ is a correction factor at wavelength λ and solar altitude h for any thickness of ozone χ.

The interpolation function $A(\lambda, h)$ is given by

$$A(\lambda, h) = \exp\{\ln[G(\lambda, h_i, 0.32)] + S(h - h_i)\}, \tag{2.4}$$

where h lies between h_i and h_{i+1}. The h_i are the six tabulated values of solar altitude, i.e. 5°, 10°, 20°, 40°, 60° and 90° for $i = 1$–6. Values of the function $G(\lambda, h, \chi)$ will be undefined for h less than 5°.

The gradient S is simply given as

$$S = \{\ln[G(\lambda, h_{i+1}, 0.32)] - \ln[G(\lambda, h_i, 0.32)]\}/(h_{i+1} - h_i). \tag{2.5}$$

The correction factor, $F(\lambda, h, \chi)$, is discussed in § 2.1.2.4.

2.1.2.2. The solar altitude *h*. It has been shown that sin h may be written as

$$\sin h = \cos \Phi \cos \delta \cos \beta + \sin \Phi \sin \delta, \tag{2.6}$$

where Φ is the geographical latitude, δ is the solar declination and β is the solar hour angle. The solar declination varies only with the day of the year, d, (January 1st = day 1, and so on) and may be calculated from

$$\delta = \arcsin(0.3978 \sin \xi), \tag{2.7}$$

where the ecliptic longitude of the Earth in its orbit ξ is obtained as a function of the day of year from the approximation

$$\xi = \omega(d - 80) + 2e[\sin(\omega d) - \sin(\omega 80)], \tag{2.8}$$

where $\omega = 2\pi/365$ and e is the eccentricity of the Earth's orbit about the Sun ($e = 0.01675$).

The solar hour angle is given in degrees by

$$\beta = 15(t - t_{sn}), \tag{2.9}$$

where t is the time of day expressed on a 24 hour clock and t_{sn} is the time of the solar noon. It follows from the above equations that given the time of day t, day of year d and geographical latitude Φ, the solar altitude h may readily be calculated.

2.1.2.3 The ozone layer thickness χ. The total amount of atmospheric ozone varies with season, latitude and longitude. Values of the average total amounts of ozone around each latitude circle of the northern hemisphere are given in table 2.2 for the seasons; winter (December, January, February), spring (March, April, May) summer (June, July, August) and autumn (September, October, November). The value which most closely approximates the day of year and latitude is selected from the table. It is not necessary to interpolate between these values since 10% variations in the expected average ozone amount are not uncommon.

Table 2.2 Mean total amount of atmospheric ozone (in cm at STP) around each latitude circle for the northern hemisphere according to London (1963).

Latitude	Winter	Spring	Summer	Autumn
0°	0.241	0.260	0.256	0.244
10°	0.247	0.268	0.261	0.253
20°	0.260	0.287	0.273	0.261
30°	0.284	0.313	0.292	0.270
40°	0.318	0.352	0.314	0.281
50°	0.357	0.395	0.333	0.299
60°	0.373	0.419	0.346	0.308
70°	0.370	0.430	0.349	0.307
80°	0.364	0.435	0.347	0.299
90°	0.361	0.436	0.339	0.290

2.1.2.4 The function $F(\lambda, h, \chi)$. This function has been empirically derived from the data presented by Bener (1972) and is not meant to represent mathematically any physical phenomenon.

It has been found that the function may adequately be represented by

$$F(\lambda, h, \chi) = \exp[-\mu(\chi - 0.32)Q], \tag{2.10}$$

where

$$\mu = \exp[0.135(320 - \lambda) - 0.4345]. \tag{2.11}$$

The parameter Q is given by either

$$Q = 1.0 \text{ for } \lambda \geqslant 330 \text{ nm} \tag{2.12}$$

or

$$Q = 1.0 + r\exp(-h/10) \cdot (h/5)^p \text{ for } \lambda < 330 \text{ nm}. \qquad (2.13)$$

The value of r may be calculated as

$$r = [7.6 - 0.35(320 - \lambda)] \exp(p) \cdot (2p)^{-p}, \qquad (2.14)$$

where

$$p = 0.6 \exp[0.06(320 - \lambda)]. \qquad (2.15)$$

2.1.2.5 Accuracy of the equations. From the equations derived above and the data given in tables 2.1 and 2.2 it is possible to compute the spectral distribution of global UVR for any desired values of t, d and Φ. The validity of the method has been checked by calculating the values of $G(\lambda, h, \chi)$ for values of χ other than 0.32 cm ozone and comparing

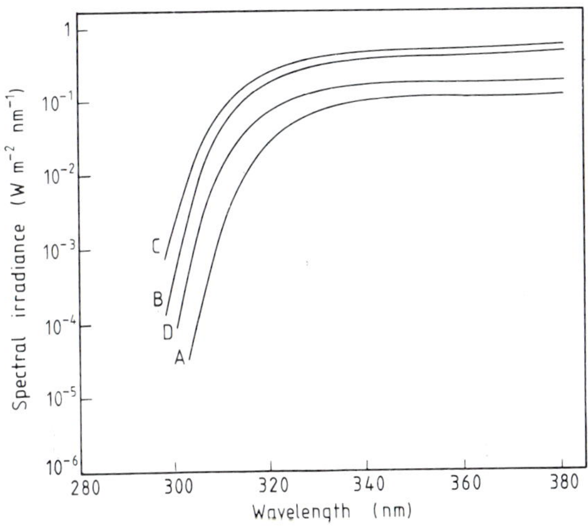

Figure 2.4 The spectral irradiance of global UVR at a latitude of 53°N on a horizontal surface at sea level at solar noon (after Diffey 1977).

Curve	Date	Solar altitude	Ozone thickness at STP (cm)
A	January 21	17°	0.357
B	April 21	49°	0.395
C	July 21	57°	0.333
D	October 21	26°	0.299

the result with the corresponding entry in Bener's tables. It has been possible to compare 450 values in this way and it was found that the average percentage deviation between the results calculated by the present method and those given by Bener was 3.7 ± 6.9% (sd), with 202 of the 450 comparisons agreeing to better than 1%. This agreement is considered to be satisfactory, since Bener estimates the errors on his values of global intensity to be in the region of 20%.

This set of equations has been used to calculate the clear-day UVR as might apply to the UK Midlands (latitude 53°N) for the four seasons at solar noon. The computed global UV spectral irradiances are shown in figure 2.4, where it may be seen that wavelengths in the region 300–315 nm (the sunburn region) are about 100 times more intense in the summer than in the winter.

2.2 The Artificial Production of UVR

2.2.1 Incandescence

A body heated to a high temperature radiates as a result of its constituent particles becoming excited by numerous interactions and collisions. For a perfect black body the power radiated at any wavelength from unit surface area of such a body is determined solely by its temperature, in accordance wth Planck's law, which is

$$M_{e\lambda} = A/\{\lambda^5[\exp(B/\lambda T) - 1]\}, \qquad (2.16)$$

where $M_{e\lambda}$ is the spectral radiant exitance at wavelength λ, T is the absolute temperature of the radiator, and A and B are constants.

As the temperature is raised, not only does the maximum power radiated increase rapidly, but the peak of the emission curve $\lambda_{\max}$ moves to a shorter wavelength, given by Wien's displacement law as

$$\lambda_{\max} = 2.898 \times 10^6/T(\mathrm{K})\ \mathrm{nm}. \qquad (2.17)$$

The Sun, of course, is the most celebrated source of incandescent UVR, although artificial incandescent sources are not efficient emitters of UVR; the ultraviolet emission from a general-purpose tungsten filament lamp is only 0.08% of the rated power for a 40 W lamp, rising to 0.1% for a 100 W lamp and 0.17% for a 1 kW lamp. However some tungsten–halogen lamps, which operate at a colour temperature of around 3000 K, may emit sufficient quantities of UVR, particularly UV-A, for applications which demand miniature optics and stable light output combined with no requirement for a high UV irradiance.

2.2.2 Gas discharges

In a discharge tube, across which there is an electric field, the electrons drift towards the anode and the positive ions towards the cathode. In a low-pressure discharge (~400 $N\,m^{-2}$) such as occurs in a fluorescent lamp, for example, one of three events may take place when a free electron collides with a neutral gas atom: the electron may undergo an elastic collision; the atom may be excited; or the atom may be ionised. In a fluorescent lamp containing a mixture of mercury and argon, the mercury is preferentially ionised since its ionisation potential (10.4 eV) is lower than that of argon (15.7 eV). The inert gases present in most practical discharge lamps act to reduce ion losses to the wall by ambipolar diffusion, control the mobility of the electrons, provide easier breakdown at a lower striking voltage and prolong the life of the electrodes by reducing sputtering and evaporation.

For a discharge to operate in a steady condition the rate of ionisation must exactly balance the rate of loss of electrons and ions by ambipolar diffusion to the walls. The consequence of this is that there is no simple relationship between voltage and current. The electrical characteristic of the discharge is very complex and dependent on all the constituents of the discharge and conditions of operation. In general, the discharge has a 'falling characteristic': the volt–ampere curve has a negative slope.

Most of the radiation from the majority of discharge lamps is from the positive column, i.e. the large uniform region of the discharge between the electrodes. The energetic electrons which produce the ionisation also produce excitation of the gas atoms, which subsequently radiate at their characteristic frequencies. Figure 2.5 shows a few of the excitation and radiating transitions in lamps containing mercury vapour.

As the pressure in a discharge tube is raised to a few atmospheres, two principal changes occur:

(a) the gas temperature increases due to the increasing number of collisions (mainly elastic collisions) with the energetic electrons;

(b) the high temperature becomes localised at the centre of the discharge, there now being a temperature gradient towards the walls, which are much cooler.

The wall becomes much less important at high pressures, and not altogether essential: discharges can operate between two electrodes

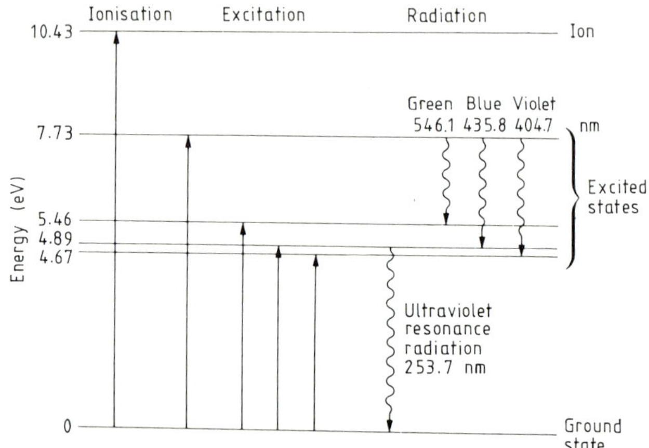

Figure 2.5 A simplified energy transition diagram for mercury (from Henderson and Marsden 1972).

without any restraining wall, and are then referred to as arcs. At high pressures the characteristic lines present in the low-pressure discharge spectrum broaden and are accompanied by a low-amplitude continuous spectrum.

2.3 Ultraviolet Radiation Lamps used in Medicine

The most common artificial sources of UVR used in medicine are mercury discharge lamps, used with or without a fluorescent coating; mercury-vapour arcs operating at various pressures; metal halide lamps; and the xenon arc lamp. This section will discuss the optical performance of these types of lamps, while the medical applications of the UVR produced by the lamps will be covered in Chapter 6.

2.3.1 Germicidal lamp

This type of lamp consists of a fused silica or Vycor (96% silica) tube filled with argon at about 1 $N\,m^{-2}$ and containing a drop of mercury. A tungsten wire electrode coated with a thermionic emitter is sealed into each end of the tube. More than 90% of the radiant energy produced by this low-pressure mercury discharge occurs at a wavelength of 254 nm (*see* figure 2.6). The remaining radiant energy is distributed among the

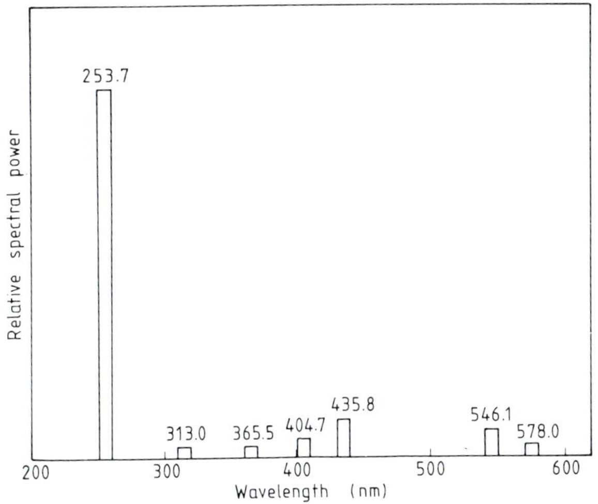

Figure 2.6 The spectral power distribution of a low-pressure mercury discharge lamp (germicidal lamp).

mercury lines in the UV-B, UV-A and visible regions which give the lamp a pale blue glow when operating.

The principal use of these lamps in medicine is for sterilisation of air and water, since the 254 nm radiation is efficient in preventing the growth of moulds and bacteria. However, 254 nm is a highly reactive wavelength to the eyes and skin (*see* Chapter 5) and for this reason these lamps should not be viewed directly.

2.3.2 Fluorescent lamps

A fluorescent lamp is simply a low-pressure mercury discharge lamp which has a phosphor coating applied to the inside of the envelope. Fluorescent radiation is produced by the excitation of the phosphor by the 254 nm radiation. The spectral power distribution of the fluorescent radiation will be a property of the chemical nature of the phosphor material. The exact chemical composition of a phosphor will depend upon the desired spectral power distribution, but essentially phosphors consist of mixtures of silicates, borates and phosphates of alkaline earth metals.

2.3.2.1 Effect of supply voltage on output. Fluctuations in the supply voltage will cause variations in lamp voltage, current, power and in the radiation output. In general a 10% increase in supply voltage will result in an 8% increase in light output on a 240 V lagging switch-start circuit but only a 4% increase in light output on a 240 V leading switch-start circuit. The variations are smaller in the leading circuit due to the presence of a capacitor.

2.3.2.2 Effect of operating temperature on output. Most fluorescent lamps yield maximum radiation output at a lamp envelope temperature of about 40 °C. This temperature is maintained when a lamp is running in free air at an ambient temperature of 25 °C. At these temperatures the vapour pressure of the mercury in the lamp is at an optimum for the production of the 254 nm radiation. As the temperature of the lamp increases, the vapour pressure also increases, which results in increased self-absorption of the resonance 254 nm radiation.

This problem can be particularly severe in irradiation units which incorporate large numbers of fluorescent lamps packed closely together, e.g. so-called PUVA units (*see* § 2.3.2.5). With standard lamps the loss in light output can be as much as 30%. To minimise the problem, fluorescent lamps are available in which a ring of indium is applied to

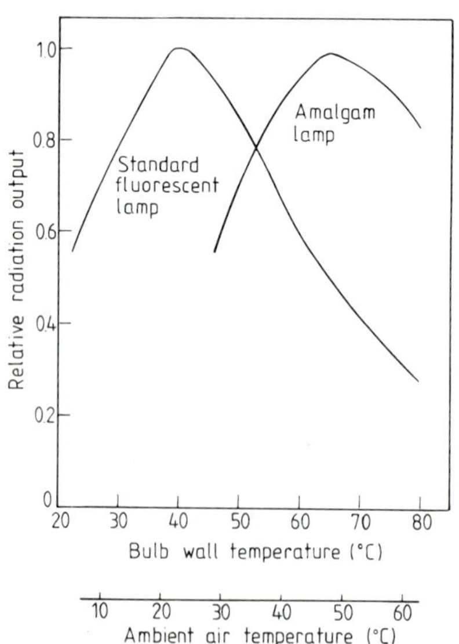

Figure 2.7 The relative radiation output for a standard fluorescent lamp and an amalgam lamp as a function of temperature.

the inside of the lamp. This forms an amalgam with the mercury when the lamp is in operation and so reduces the vapour pressure. Although these lamps operate at maximum efficiency at temperatures above normal, giving gains in radiation output at those temperatures of up to 25%, their output will be less than that of the standard fluorescent lamp when run at normal ambient temperatures. The relative radiation output for a standard fluorescent lamp and a typical amalgam lamp is shown as a function of lamp envelope temperature and ambient air temperature in figure 2.7. Although the amalgam lamp is theoretically more desirable in irradiation systems which generate a large amount of heat, economic considerations have prevented their use in some commercially available whole-body (PUVA) irradiation units and instead manufacturers prefer to rely upon forced-air cooling to maintain the lamp envelope at a suitable temperature.

2.3.2.3 The life of fluorescent lamps. A fluorescent lamp normally fails when the emissive material on the cathodes ceases to produce sufficient electrons to permit the lamp to strike. A sign of a lamp nearing the end of its useful life is severe blackening at both ends of the tube. The light output of a fluorescent tube designed for general lighting purposes falls by about 2–4% during its first 100 h of life and thereafter at a slower rate until at 2000 h it has fallen by only a further 5–10%. However, UV fluorescent lamps have phosphors which are less stable than those used in general lighting lamps and the radiation output shows a more rapid degradation in the first 100 h, with the lamp restricted to a useful life of about 1000 h.

2.3.2.4 The fluorescent sunlamp. This low-pressure mercury discharge lamp incorporates a phosphor coated onto the inside of the lamp envelope which results in a continuous spectrum from about 270–380 nm with a peak at 313 nm (*see* figure 2.8). Note also in this figure the presence of the mercury characteristic lines superimposed on the continuum and present also in the visible region. These lines are present in all mercury fluorescent lamps irrespective of the phosphor material. However, it is possible to suppress the emission of certain lines either by using a lamp envelope material which absorbs unwanted short-wavelength radiation or by incorporating a suitable filter in the lamp envelope, e.g. the 'black-light' lamp. The fluorescent sunlamp is used extensively in actinotherapy and the spectrum shown in figure 2.8 is produced by the Westinghouse FS20T12 and the Philips TL12 lamps.

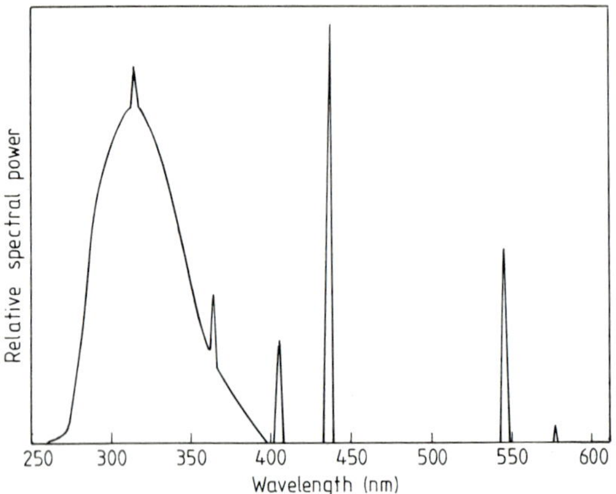

Figure 2.8 The spectral power distribution of a fluorescent sunlamp.

2.3.2.5 The fluorescent UV-A lamp. The rapid increase in the treatment of the skin disease, psoriasis, by the combination of the photoactive drug 8-methoxypsoralen and long-wave ultraviolet radiation is partially due to the advent of high-intensity fluorescent UV-A lamps. The spectral power distribution of this lamp is shown in figure 2.9 and consists of a continuum from about 315–400 nm accompanied again by the mercury lines in the UV-A and visible regions, which gives the lamp a bluish-white

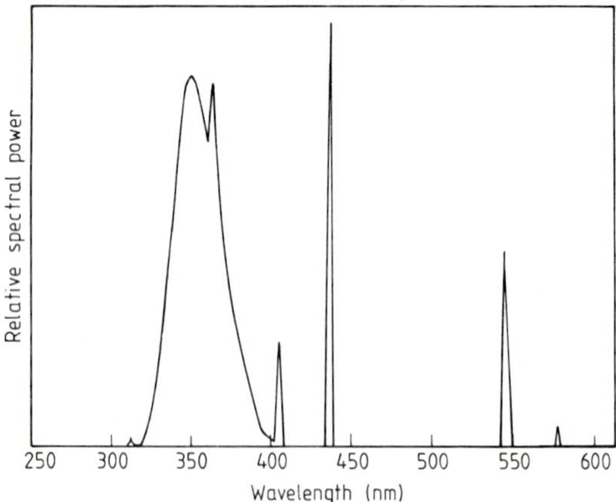

Figure 2.9 The spectral power distribution of a fluorescent UV-A lamp.

appearance when operating. The high output from this type of lamp is achieved by including a reflecting surface in the lamp itself. The first reflecting coat usually consists of titanium dioxide and extends over the length of the lamp and about 225° around the circumference. The whole lamp is then coated with the phosphor layer on top of the reflecting layer so that the reflecting layer is sandwiched between the phosphor and the lamp envelope. These lamps are 10–15% less efficient than the standard fluorescent lamp but have about 50% more radiation directed in the forward direction. This is a great advantage when the lamps are packed tightly together in the cylindrical geometry of a whole-body UV irradiation unit as illustrated in figure 6.3 (*see* p 114) and results in a reasonably uniform UV-A irradiance of the order of 50–100 $\mathrm{W\,m^{-2}}$ at the patient's skin.

2.3.2.6 The 'black-light' lamp. The 'black-light' fluorescent lamp emits a similar spectral power distribution to the UV-A fluorescent lamp in the region 315–400 nm but with suppression of the mercury lines in the visible spectrum. This results from using a visible-absorbing, UV-A transmitting, glass envelope. When switched off the lamp envelope appears almost black. A purplish light is perceived when the lamp is operating. The black-light lamp is used for photopatch testing.

2.3.3 Mercury arc lamps

The radiation emitted from a mercury-vapour arc lamp arises from two mechanisms. Line or characteristic radiation is produced as a result of excitation of the constituent atoms together with a spectral continuum chiefly due to ion and electron recombination. When a mercury arc lamp is switched on the vapour pressure of mercury is low and a discharge fills the lamp and appears blue, with a relatively high proportion of radiated energy in the ultraviolet. As the temperature of the discharge rises, and with it the mercury vapour pressure, the radiated energy is concentrated progressively in the spectral lines of the visible region, and this, together with the introduction of a small proportion of continuous radiation, results in the discharge becoming whiter. After about 5–6 minutes the lamp is fully run-up and in the medium-pressure mercury arc lamp the mercury vapour pressure is in the range 2–10 atm (1 atm = $1.013 \times 10^5\ \mathrm{N\,m^{-2}}$) depending on the lamp rating. High-pressure mercury arc lamps operate at a pressure of 10–100 atm which results in broadening of the spectral lines and an increase in the continuum relative to the characteristic radiation. The spectral power distribution

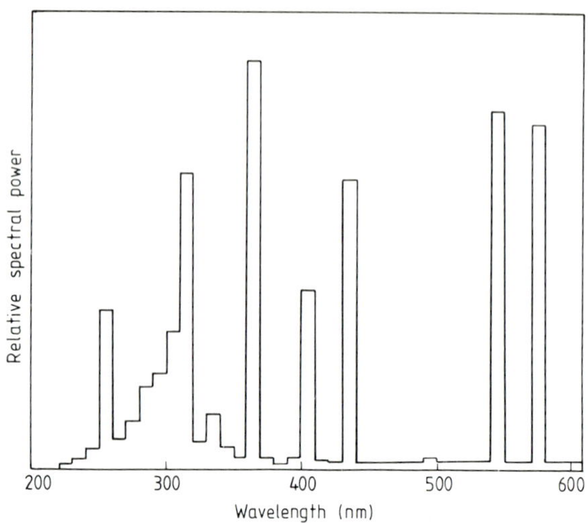

Figure 2.10 The spectral power distribution of a medium-pressure mercury arc lamp.

of a medium-pressure mercury arc lamp in a quartz envelope is shown in figure 2.10 and consists of the line spectrum of mercury with some continuous radiation.

2.3.3.1 The high-pressure mercury compact arc lamp. This is a useful lamp for the medical physics department wishing to provide a calibration facility for UV measurement devices. In the 100 W lamp the electrode spacing is of the order of 0.25 mm, resulting in a point source of light of high luminance. Also, the 365 nm mercury line can readily be isolated with colour glass filters to produce a monochromatic source of radiation in the UV-A region.

The bulb of a compact arc lamp is nearly spherical, to prevent the lamp surface becoming too hot, and fabricated from a good quality fused silica. The electrodes in the lamp are machined from tungsten rod, which may contain a small proportion, about 3%, of thoria to reduce the work function and lower the lamp starting voltage. In a compact arc lamp designed for DC operation the anode is usually larger than the cathode, since the voltage fall, and consequently the power dissipation, is higher at the anode. The luminance distribution along the discharge length is almost constant except in the regions adjacent to the electrodes, but the distribution across the discharge at its centre is approximately Gaussian. As the lamp ages the shape of the electrodes is modified by local melting and this can affect the characteristics and stability of the discharge. This is accompanied by deterioration of the thoriated tungsten electrodes and the bulb progressively darkens due to tungsten evaporation, resulting in reduced light output.

2.3.3.2 The Alpine sunlamp. The Alpine sunlamp is probably the most common source of UVR found in physiotherapy departments. It is designed for general or regional irradiation of individual patients.

The source of UVR in the Alpine sunlamp is a U-shaped medium-pressure mercury arc lamp with an envelope designed not to emit ozone producing radiation, i.e. UVR of wavelengths less than 270 nm. The lamp is positioned at the approximate focus of a paraboloid anodised alu-

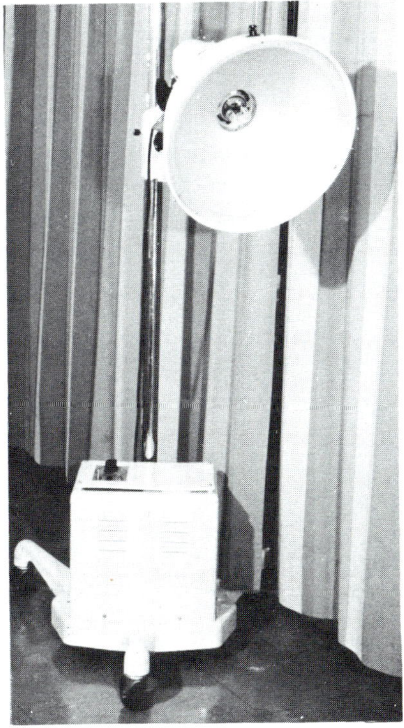

Figure 2.11 The Alpine sunlamp.

minium reflector in order to produce a high degree of spatial uniformity over the treatment area. The lamp and reflector are mounted on a vertical shaft which incorporates a counterbalanced rise and fall system. Pivot points permit angular adjustment of the lamp housing in all planes. At the base of the unit is the lamp power supply. The deterioration in lamp output during the life of the lamp can be approximately compensated by increasing the lamp power at infrequent intervals. This adjustment of lamp power with use serves to maintain a reasonably constant output. A photograph of the Alpine sunlamp is shown in figure 2.11.

2.3.3.3 The Kromayer lamp. Another lamp used by physiotherapists is the Kromayer lamp shown in figure 2.12. It is designed principally for contact therapy but can also be used with applicators for irradiation of body cavities. The source of UVR is again a medium-pressure mercury arc, but in a quartz envelope to permit the bactericidal UV-C radiation to be emitted. In order to allow contact therapy, the outer window is kept cool by circulating water. It is important to use distilled water as the coolant to minimise the presence of impurities, such as dissolved

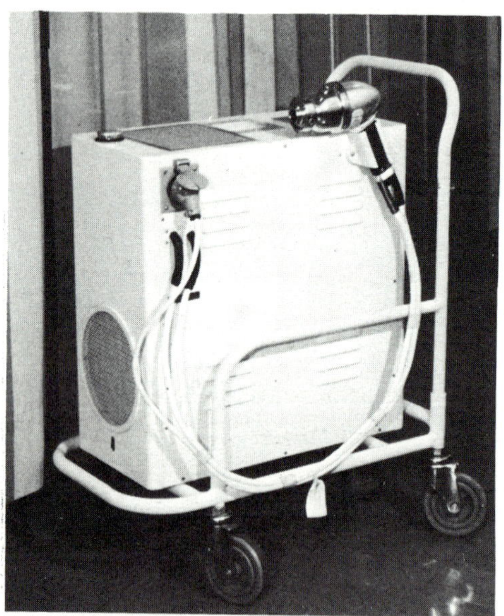

Figure 2.12 The Kromayer lamp.

salts, which can grossly attenuate UV-B and UV-C. For the same reason the outer window should be cleaned regularly.

2.3.3.4 The Wood's lamp. This lamp, named after its inventor R W Wood, is essentially a source of UV-A commonly used by dermatologists for the diagnosis of various disorders by employing the phenomenon of fluorescence. Basically, the unit consists of a medium-pressure mercury arc mounted behind a UV-A transmitting, visible-light absorbing, glass filter, commonly known as 'black glass' or 'Wood's glass'. Wood's original design in 1903 used a nickel oxide glass filter. Modern Wood's lamps may probably incorporate a filter of different chemical composition, but they are all essentially monochromatic sources of 365 nm radiation with little intensity at the other mercury wavelengths in either the UV or visible regions.

2.3.4 Metal halide lamps

In a high-pressure mercury lamp a considerable volume of the arc tube is not effectively used to emit radiation. This non-productive space is required to reduce energy dissipation at the wall of the arc tube in order to maintain a long lamp life. If, however, another element of low excitation potential can be introduced without interfering unduly with the mercury discharge, then this element can be excited in the otherwise non-productive space, resulting in additional output and spectral content. The most common added elements are the alkali metals, used in the alkali metal iodide form to eliminate chemical attack on the silica envelope.

The inclusion of metal halides in discharge lamps provides a significant gain in UV output compared to ordinary mercury arc lamps; a metal halide lamp of 1800 W emits about 22% of its radiation at wavelengths less than 400 nm. The spectral power distribution depends, of course, on the particular metal halide. Lamps which contain halides of gallium and of dysprosium, as well as mercury, have been employed as UV sources for irradiation of patients with psoriasis. In general, though, metal halide lamps have been primarily developed for the graphic art industry and so far have found little application in medicine.

2.3.5 Xenon arc lamps

In the xenon arc the radiation is emitted primarily as a continuum, unlike the mercury arc which essentially emits a line spectrum. The production of the continuum is optimum under conditions of high specific power, high current density and high internal pressure, leading to compact, bright sources. Because of high operating temperatures the lamp envelope is normally constructed from fused silica. Xenon lamps consist of an arc burning between solid tungsten electrodes in a pressure of pure xenon and may be designed to operate from AC or DC. Cold-filling pressures up to 12 atm are commonly used and as a result there exists a potential hazard from explosive failure of the lamp, although in practice lamp explosions are rare. The lamps can be of the compact form, when the bulb is nearly spherical, or the linear form which utilises a cylindrical lamp envelope. The compact xenon arc lamp is available in power ratings from 75 W to 25 kW or more. Linear source lamps of up to 65 kW are used for floodlighting in sports stadia. Because xenon lamps contain a permanent gas filling, the full radiation output is available immediately after switching on; there is no run-up period as in arc lamps containing mercury which has to vaporise.

The spectral power distribution of the xenon arc lamp is shown in figure 2.13. Because of the similarity of the spectrum to that of the solar spectrum (*see* figure 2.1), the xenon lamp has been employed as a laboratory source of sunlight, the so-called solar simulator. Also because of its continuous spectrum the xenon lamp is commonly used in conjunction with a monochromator for biological action spectrum studies.

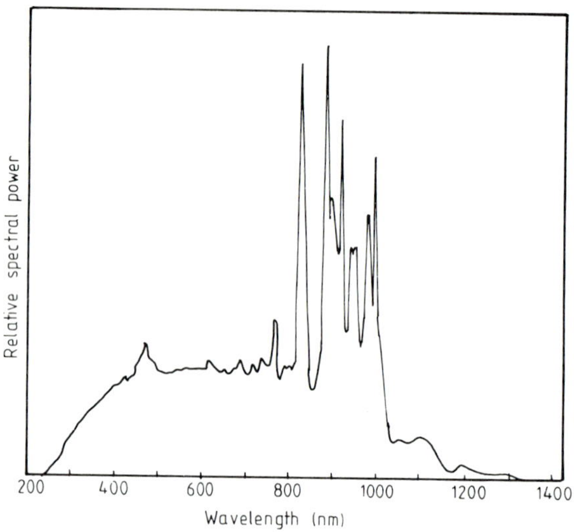

Figure 2.13 The spectral power distribution of a xenon arc lamp.

A detailed description of the clinical irradiation monochromator is given in Chapter 3.

2.3.5.1 The solar simulator. The ultraviolet component of sunlight is responsible for most light induced skin reactions and so any artificial source designed to elicit various normal and pathological photoresponses should produce a spectral power distribution similar to that of sunlight in the range 290–400 nm. An instrument which fulfills this criterion, the so-called solar simulator, utilises a high-pressure xenon arc lamp used in conjunction with collecting and focusing optics and spectral shaping filters.

The specification and design of a solar UV simulator has been described by Berger (1969). In this system the optical components are selected such that the spectral power distribution produced by the simulator resembles the spectral distribution of global UVR as measured at a latitude of 41°N in the summer at midday, i.e. a solar altitude of 70°. The optical design of a typical solar simulator comprises a 150 W xenon lamp, quartz lenses, a dichroic mirror to reduce the infrared component, a Schott WG320 colour glass filter to provide a short wavelength cutoff in the region of 295 nm and a Corning 9863 'black glass' filter which approximates the desired long-wave ultraviolet cutoff.

A uniform area 1 cm in diameter is produced at the focal point in front of the exit aperture and results in an irradiance at this point of 750 W m^{-2}, of which 520 W m^{-2} is at wavelengths below 400 nm. The time required to produce a minimal erythema (sunburn) is about three minutes.

3 Optical Components

It is often required in photobiological studies that a radiation beam be focused, reflected, dispersed or filtered. Indeed, one of the most common tools in photobiology, the irradiation monochromator, may incorporate all of these features. In this chapter discussion on optical components will be biased towards factors affecting practical usage, as it is assumed that the reader is already familiar with the theoretical aspects of geometrical optics.

3.1 Lenses

3.1.1 Lens material

In general, optical lenses are made from crown glass. However, since the transmission of UVR through crown glass drops rapidly as the wavelength decreases below about 350 nm, lenses for use in the ultraviolet are normally constructed from fused silica. Optical-quality synthetic fused silica lenses are ideally suited for applications in the UV-A and UV-B, although their transmission diminishes in the UV-C. Nevertheless,

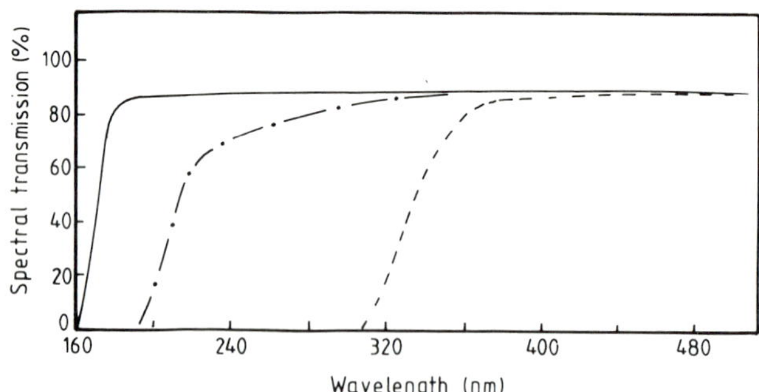

Figure 3.1 The spectral transmission (including surface reflections) of optical crown glass (broken curve), optical quality synthetic fused silica (chain curve) and suprasil (full curve). Each material is 10 mm in thickness (from Melles Griot 1975, with permission).

it is possible to obtain high-quality synthetic fused silica ('suprasil') which has a high transmission down to about 180 nm. A comparison of the spectral transmission of optical crown glass, optical quality synthetic fused silica and suprasil is shown in figure 3.1.

Synthetic fused silica (amorphous silicon dioxide) is formed by the chemical combination of silicon and oxygen and should not be confused with fused quartz which is made by crushing and melting natural crystals. Synthetic fused silica is far purer than natural materials. This increased purity assures higher UV transmission, improved homogeneity and freedom from striae or inclusions.

3.1.2 Types of lens

3.1.2.1 Convex lenses. Both plano–convex and bi-convex lenses conventionally have positive focal lengths, converge incident light and form both real and virtual images. The convex lens is probably the most widely-used lens in photobiology and is generally employed as the input optics in an irradiation monochromator to form an image of the source at the entrance slit of the monochromator. This can be achieved by using a single bi-convex lens between the radiation source and the monochromator, or, for maximum efficiency in transferring radiation from the source to the entrance slit, pairs of plano–convex lenses can be used in the convex-side-facing-convex-side orientation.

3.1.2.2 Concave lenses. Both plano–concave and bi-concave lenses conventionally have negative focal lengths, diverge collimated incident light and form only virtual images which are seen through the lens. Concave lenses find little application in photobiology.

3.1.2.3 Cylindrical lenses. Cylindrical lenses are used in applications requiring magnification along one axis only, such as changing the width of an image without changing its height. The standard cylindrical lenses are plano–convex in form and rectangular in shape. They are useful for photobiological work in modifying the long, thin image at the exit slit of a monochromator to one of a more square cross section, which is better suited for patient irradiation in action spectrum studies.

3.2 Mirrors

3.2.1 Mirror substrates and coatings

Substrate materials for mirrors include optical crown glass, optical-quality borosilicate and optical-quality synthetic fused silica. Optical crown glass is preferable when economy is a major constraint, while borosilicate and synthetic fused silica are preferred in applications demanding thermal stability and reliability in flatness specifications. The coefficients of linear thermal expansion of optical crown glass, Pyrex and synthetic fused silica are approximately 9×10^{-6}, 3.2×10^{-6} and $0.5 \times 10^{-6}\ K^{-1}$ respectively.

Because of the transmission characteristics of optical crown glass and Pyrex in the ultraviolet it is essential that mirrors are coated on the front surface. Aluminium is the most widely used material for coating mirrors and offers consistently high reflectance throughout the near-infrared, visible and UV-A.

By applying a film of an ultraviolet-transmitting dielectric (usually MgF_2), the reflectivity of pure, bare aluminium can be preserved and enhanced throughout the UV-B and UV-C. The dielectric layer prevents oxidation of the aluminium surface and provides abrasion resistance. Reflectance averages over 88% from 180–400 nm, and over 85% throughout the visible. Silver should never be used for UV-reflecting mirrors for two reasons:

(a) its reflectance drops off rapidly for wavelengths below 360 nm, falling to about 10% at 300 nm, and

(b) as a front-surface coating, silver readily oxidises, which results in tarnishing.

3.2.2 Types of mirror

3.2.2.1 Concave spherical reflectors. Concave spherical reflectors normally consist of an optical crown glass substrate with a front-surface coating of UV-enhanced aluminium. They are often used to increase the light output of illumination systems by increasing the efficiency with which light sources are utilised. For this purpose the reflector is located with its centre of curvature coinciding with the source. Concave spherical reflectors are usually employed as the collimating and telescope mirrors in monochromators. These mirrors are located such that the centre of curvature coincides with the entrance and exit slits respectively and results in a parallel beam of radiation being transmitted to and received from the dispersing element.

3.2.2.2 Paraboloidal and ellipsoidal reflectors. Concave paraboloidal and ellipsoidal reflectors are the basis for a variety of high-efficiency illumination, light collection and light concentration systems. The high collection efficiency follows from the fundamental geometrical properties of the parabola and ellipse.

These reflectors may be fabricated from optical crown glass either by conventional grinding and polishing or by an electrolytic replication process which very accurately reproduces the geometry and finish of a carefully generated master surface. Replication begins with electrolytic deposition of a nickel substrate, the thickness of which is designed and controlled to achieve desired mechanical properties. Upon separation from the master the nickel substrate is electrolytically coated with a highly reflective yet extremely hard and durable rhodium film.

An ellipsoidal reflector can be used in an irradiation monochromator as an essentially complete condenser; the source is placed at one focus of the ellipse and the entrance slit at the other focus, thus eliminating the need for a condensing lens.

3.3 Optical Filters

Optical filters are used, in general, to suppress unwanted wavelengths from the radiation source reaching the object, whilst at the same time allowing the desirable spectral region to irradiate the object with the minimum of attenuation. There are many types of optical filter although this section will limit itself to a description of some of the more common filters.

3.3.1 Heat-absorbing filters

This type of filter is used to reduce localised temperatures to acceptable values in illumination systems. For example heat-absorbing filters can usefully be situated in the light path between an arc lamp and the entrance slit of a monochromator in order to reduce damage to the internal optical components of the monochromator. The control of heat from a radiation source can be achieved in one of two ways. The infrared can be separated from the rest of the emission spectrum either by blocking infrared from places where it is unwanted, or diverting it to places from which the resulting heat may be readily dissipated.

Heat blocking, or absorption, can be achieved by means of either an infrared opaque glass or a fused silica cell containing distilled water which combines high transmission for ultraviolet down to about 200 nm with good attenuation in selected wavebands in the infrared region. Water exhibits high transmission in the infrared (so called 'infrared windows') in the following wavelength intervals: the visible region to 1.3 μm, 1.5–1.8 μm, 2.0–2.5 μm, 3.4–4.2 μm and 8–13 μm. There is negligible transmission of infrared radiation through water at wavelengths greater than 15 μm. The xenon arc lamp, which is commonly used as a light source in photobiology, has a high radiant power emission in the spectral interval 800–1000 nm (1 μm) (*see* figure 2.13). This emission corresponds to one of the 'infrared windows' and consequently water is a poor medium for effective attenuation of this component in the near infrared. The presence of dissolved salts or of organic matter in water affects the transmission in the ultraviolet region profoundly and so if the water is recirculated through a closed system, e.g. as in the Kromayer lamp (*see* § 2.3.3.3), it is important to renew the water at frequent intervals.

Figure 3.2 shows the internal transmittance of some Schott heat-absorbing filters, 2 mm in thickness. Unfortunately the transmittance drops rapidly at wavelengths below about 350 nm and for this reason this type of filter is not suitable when significant intensities of UV-B and UV-C are required.

The diversion of heat is based upon a spectrally selective reflector (hot or cold mirror) utilising multilayer thin-film principles. This type of mirror, often called a 'dichroic mirror', can be maximised for reflection

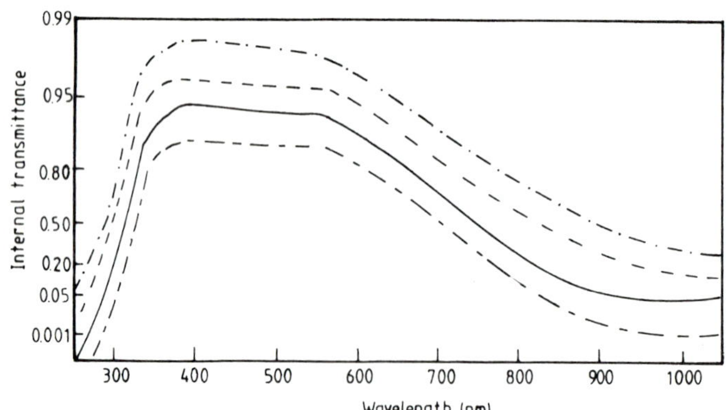

Figure 3.2 Internal transmittance of 2 mm thick Schott heat-absorbing glass filters (with permission from Jenaer Glaswerk Schott & Gen, Mainz, West Germany).

in the desired spectral region, whilst at the same time transmitting most of the unwanted radiation (cold mirror); or, alternatively, heat may be reflected and the desired radiation transmitted (hot mirror). For example, dichroic mirrors exist which have 99% reflectance of UV-A combined with about 10% reflectance over much of the visible and infrared. Unfortunately a dichroic mirror is usually a very expensive means of removing heat from a system and may be as much as 30 times the cost of a heat-absorbing glass filter. For this reason its use is limited in clinical photobiology.

3.3.2 Neutral-density filters

Neutral-density filters allow attenuation of the radiation beam without a significant change in chromaticity. They are useful in attenuating high-intensity beams to levels at which the detection device is more accurate and linear, thereby extending the useful range of the instrument. The irradiance of the unattenuated beam can then be calculated from the known optical density of the filter. Optical density (D) is defined as the base 10 logarithm of the reciprocal of transmittance (T) and is expressed as

$$D = \log_{10}(1/T) \tag{3.1}$$

or

$$T = 10^{-D}. \tag{3.2}$$

The definition of optical density is analogous to the definition of decibel as used in electronics. Good-quality neutral-density filters consist of a thin film of metallic alloy on an optical-grade synthetic fused silica substrate and can attenuate from 200–2500 nm with a high degree of linearity.

Since neutral density filters are not strictly independent of wavelength in their attenuation, it is advisable to calibrate them over the range of wavelengths to be used, for work requiring high accuracy.

3.3.3 Absorption filters

Absorption, or colour glass, filters are widely used either singly or in combination with other types of filter, for isolating different regions of the electromagnetic spectrum from 200 nm–3 μm. Glass absorption filters are cheap and commercially available in sizes from 10 mm in diameter up to 0.6 m square and from 1–10 mm in thickness. The transmission properties of a filter are dependent upon the glass base; the absorbing material, or colourant, dispersed in the base; and frequently on the thermal treatment of the filter. Typical base glasses are potassium, sodium, phosphate, borate, borosilicate and silicate. The colourants may take the form of metal ions in solution in the base glass, e.g., Ti, V, Cr, Mn, Fe, Co, Ni, Cu, Y, Zr, Mo, La, Ce, Pr, Nd, W and U. Alternatively, they may consist of metal atoms—e.g., Au, Ag, Cu and Pt—or of non-metallic elements or their compounds—e.g., S, sulphides, Se, selenides, Te and P—that are suspended in the glass in the form of submicroscopic crystals that reach their active size only after a special heat treatment called striking. Finally, the colouration of the filter may be due to the base glass alone.

3.3.3.1 Transmittance curves of glass absorption filters. There are something like 13 major manufacturers of glass filters mainly based in either the USA, Germany or Japan. Unfortunately, however, the various manufacturers present information on the spectral transmittance of their filters in a variety of ways. Some present their data in tabular, others in graphical form. Transmittance, log (transmittance), optical density or log (optical density) may be plotted along the ordinate axis. Also the transmittances or optical densities may refer to internal or to external values, which take into account reflection losses at the filter surfaces.

The transmission curves presented here are reproduced from the Schott colour filter glass catalogue and are plotted on a log (internal optical density) scale. The advantages of plotting the data in this way are:

(a) the shape of the curve depends only on the spectral absorption coefficient of the filter. Changes in the concentration of the colourant or in the thickness of the filter are equivalent to a relative vertical displacement of the curve and the ordinate scale;

(b) the log (internal optical density) scale is almost linear in the 0.05–0.80 transmittance regions, but expands both the low- and the high-transmittance regions revealing details that would otherwise be lost if a linear or log (transmittance) scale were used.

For most glass filters the external transmittance is approximately equal to the internal transmittance multiplied by 0.915 for all wavelengths from 220 nm–2.5 μm. The factor 0.915 takes into account reflection losses for both faces of the glass filter and is calculated from Fresnel's laws of reflection using a refractive index of 1.52.

The most common type of glass absorption filter is the short-wavelength cut-on long-wavelength pass filter. At wavelengths less than the so-called cut-on spectral region the transmission falls rapidly and, in general, the greater the rate of fall of transmission with decreasing wavelength, the more useful is the filter. These filters are available with a cut-on wavelength from 220–780 nm in steps of 10–20 nm. Figure 3.3 shows the internal transmittance curves of Schott filters of 1 mm in thickness with cut-on wavelengths in the ultraviolet region of the electromagnetic spectrum.

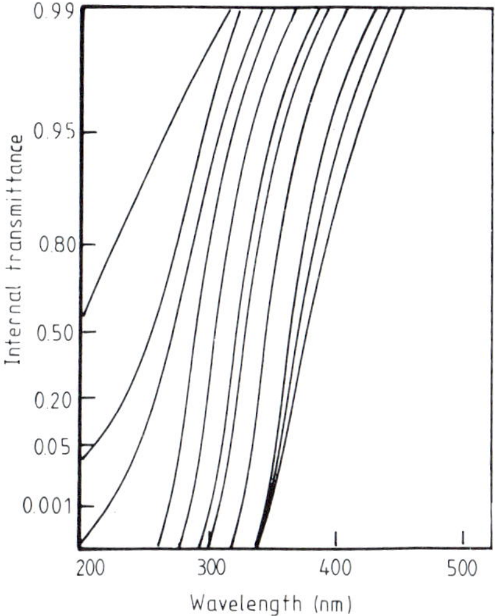

Figure 3.3 Internal transmittance of Schott glass filters (1 mm thick) with cut-on wavelengths in the ultraviolet (with permission from Jenaer Glaswerk Schott & Gen, Mainz, West Germany).

A useful filter for selective transmission in the ultraviolet combined with high absorption of visible radiation is the so-called ultraviolet transmitting black-glass filter. The Schott UG1 filter, whose internal transmittance is shown in figure 3.4, is often used in conjunction with a photodiode to produce a UV-A detector. However, it should be noted that black glass (often referred to as Wood's glass) also transmits radiation in the near infrared, and, when used in conjunction with silicon photodiodes in particular, may result in an appreciable fraction of the detector signal being due to irradiation by infrared radiation from the source. The effect is negligible when a GaAsP photodiode is used as these devices have no infrared response (*see* figure 4.7).

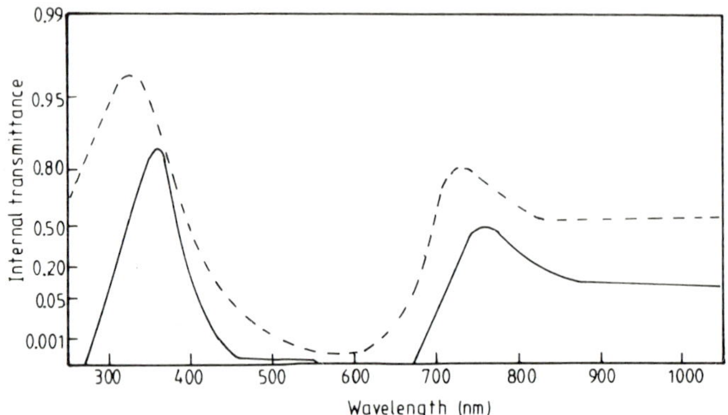

Figure 3.4 Internal transmittance of Schott ultraviolet transmitting black glass filters, 1 mm thick: full curve, UG1; broken curve, UG5. (With permission from Jenaer Glaswerk Schott & Gen, Mainz, West Germany.)

The Schott UG5 filter (*see* figure 3.4) is useful where a high transmission in the UV-B is required. To obtain a filter such as the UG5, with high transmission at shorter wavelengths, demands a high-purity glass which has a poor resistance to weathering compared to the UG1 and also exhibits changes of transmission with UV irradiation.

3.3.3.2 Factors affecting the use of glass absorption filters. Glass filters should be treated gently and care should be taken not to touch the transmitting surfaces of the filter, although they may be readily cleaned with organic solvents. On the whole the optical quality of glass filters is good, but striae and bubbles may occur during manufacture and filters should be checked for them.

The transmittance curves of short-wavelength cut-on filters are displaced to longer wavelengths with increase in temperature, with temperature coefficients varying from 0.02–0.04 nm K^{-1} for the temperature interval between 10°C and 90°C. This effect is largest in glasses that contain selenium or sulphur; for example a yellow CdS glass becomes transparent when immersed in liquid air and red on heating. Glass filters exposed to UVR often show a gradual decrease in transmission and changes in spectral transmittance, a phenomenon known as 'solarisation'.

Some glass filters may tarnish on exposure to high humidity or high temperature for prolonged periods. It is possible to overcome this by specially hardening the filter during manufacture or, alternatively, by protecting the filter either by cementing it between two stable glasses or by the deposition on it of protective quartz or other metal oxide layers.

Fluorescence in the UV and visible regions of the spectrum is exhibited by some glass filters. If this feature is undesirable the effect can be reduced by using an auxiliary filter to remove either the exciting radiation or the fluorescence itself.

In keeping with most glasses, glass absorption filters can be discoloured by high doses of ionising radiation, the amount of discolouration depending upon the base glass and the radiation dose.

3.3.4 Interference filters

An interference filter permits the transmission of a narrow band of wavelengths, whilst at the same time prohibiting the transmission of wavelengths outside the desired band. This type of filter may be regarded

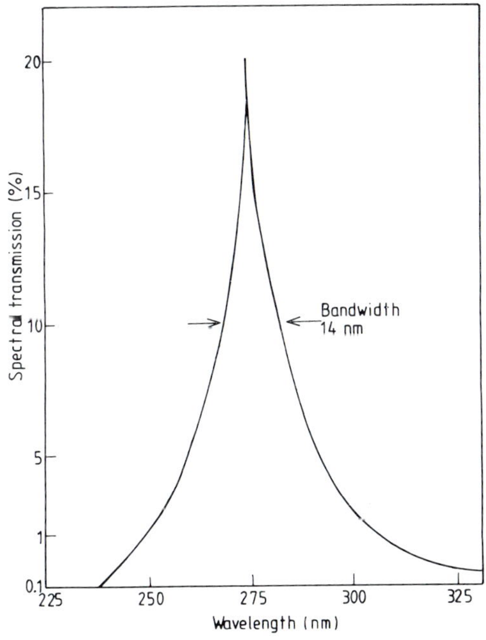

Figure 3.5 Spectral transmission curve of a typical interference filter for use in the ultraviolet.

as a classical Fabry–Perot interferometer. Interference filters are manufactured by vacuum depositing layers of a non-absorbing dielectric material of carefully controlled thickness between two partially reflecting metal layers. The thickness, t, of the dielectric layer determines the central wavelength, λ, of the transmission band since in general t is chosen such that

$$t = \lambda/2. \tag{3.3}$$

Improved performance in terms of increased rejection of unwanted wavelengths may be achieved by using dielectric multilayer stacks as reflectors. By varying the number of layers in the reflector, the bandwidth of the filter can be adjusted from less than 1 nm to about 100 nm, whilst exhibiting a transmission outside the pass band of around 10^{-7}.

The transmission curve of a typical interference filter is shown in figure 3.5.

3.3.4.1 Factors affecting performance

(1) Temperature: interference filters are generally designed for use at room temperature, although continuous operation between −50°C and +70°C is permissible. However, it should be borne in mind that the peak wavelength transmitted by the filter will shift with change in temperature due to thermal expansion (or contraction) of the layers in combination with a temperature dependant change of the refractive indices. The peak wavelength increases with temperature, and vice versa. The rate of shift is approximately linear and depends upon the peak wavelength. Typical coefficients are 0.015 nm K^{-1} at 400 nm peak, 0.018 nm K^{-1} at 656 nm peak and 0.03 nm K^{-1} at 1000 nm peak.

(2) Angle of incidence: it is clear that the transmission characteristics of an interference filter depend upon the path length of the radiation in the dielectric, and that the light path changes with angle of incidence. It is observed that the peak wavelength shifts to shorter wavelengths as the angle of incidence deviates from normal incidence. This wavelength shift is accompanied by a reduction in peak transmittance and sometimes by distortion of the transmittance curve.

The change in peak wavelength can be described as a function of angle of incidence and refractive index of the filter. For collimated radiation incident at angles up to about 10° from the normal, the peak wavelength is given by

$$\lambda_\alpha = \lambda_0 (1 - (N_e/N_f)^2 \sin^2 \alpha)^{1/2}, \tag{3.4}$$

where λ_α is the peak wavelength for an angle of incidence α; λ_0 is the peak wavelength at normal incidence; N_e is the refractive index of the external medium ($N_e = 1.0$ for air); and N_f is the refractive index of the filter ($N_f = 1.45$ for a cryolite dielectric or $N_f = 2.1$ for a zinc sulphide dielectric).

(3) Orientation of the filter: as a general rule the high reflecting (shiney or metallic looking) side of an interference filter should always face the source of radiation. This ensures that the thermal load on the filter will be minimised, as the absorbing colour glass faces away from the source and most of the unwanted radiation is reflected back. Apart from the thermal effect, the direction from which radiation enters the filters does not influence the transmittance at or near the pass band.

3.4 Irradiation Monochromators

One of the fundamental investigations in the study of how an observable effect is produced in a biological species when exposed to non-ionising radiation is the determination of the degree to which different wavelengths of radiation are able to initiate the effect. For example, which wavelengths of UVR are most effective in eliciting erythema in human skin or photokeratitis in the eye? To answer these and other questions it is necessary to irradiate the subject with monochromatic radiation of different wavelengths. The term 'monochromatic' is in fact misleading since the spectral distribution of radiation emerging from the exit slit of an irradiation monochromator is usually approximately triangular, the shape of the distribution being a function of the entrance and exit slit widths.

Most commercial UV monochromators are designed for spectroscopic use to give beams of high spectral purity but with little emphasis on high intensity. However, for photobiological work an instrument is required which will transmit a band of wavelengths from 2–10 nm wide with high intensity. Such a system typically consists of a source of UVR of high radiance used in conjunction with a monochromator incorporating one or possibly two dispersing elements. The most common radiation source for clinical photobiology is the xenon arc lamp, which has been described in the previous chapter, and so the remainder of this chapter will limit itself to a description of the design and performance of monochromators.

3.4.1 Monochromator design

A classical irradiation monochromator consists of a source of radiation, entrance optics, an entrance aperture, a collimator, a dispersing device, a telescope and an exit aperture. The basic components are illustrated in figure 3.6 in the so-called Czerny–Turner design. Light from the radiation source is used to illuminate the entrance slit S_1 placed at the focus of the collimating mirror M_1. Light is reflected from M_1 as a parallel beam and impinges on the dispersing element, which may be either a prism or a grating. The element disperses the incident radiation into its component wavelengths each as a separate bundle of parallel rays inclined at different angles to the plane of the dispersion device. Each of these bundles of rays is collected by the telescope mirror M_2 and brought to a focus in the plane of the exit slit S_2. Each wavelength in turn can be brought to S_2 by suitable rotation of the dispersing element.

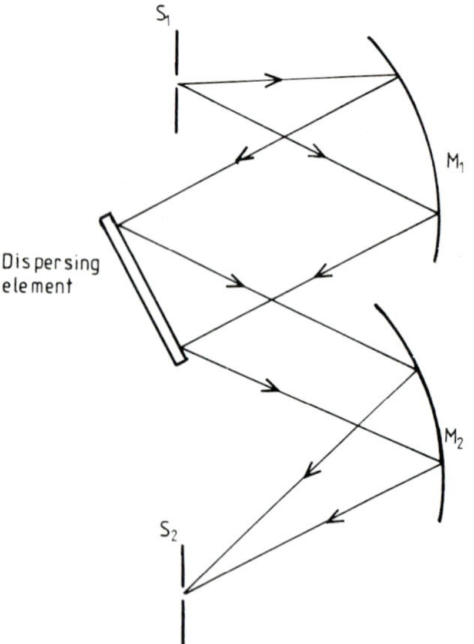

Figure 3.6 The basic components of an irradiation monochromator: S_1, entrance slit; M_1, collimating mirror; M_2 telescope mirror; and S_2 exit slit.

Some of the factors which affect the efficiency of an irradiation monochromator are discussed in the following subsections.

3.4.1.1 Illumination of the entrance slit. The usual way of illuminating the entrance slit of a monochromator is to focus the light from the source by a lens or mirror to form a real image of the source at the entrance slit. The main goal of the input optics is to put as much radiation as possible through the entrance slit within the acceptance angle of the instrument. To achieve this the diameter of the condensing lens should be large enough to completely fill the collimating mirror with light, but not to overfill it, since this only serves to increase unwanted stray light which finds its way to the exit slit.

Since there are unavoidable reflection and transmission losses in the condensing lens, it may be wondered why the source is not put directly at the entrance slit. The reason is that generally the entrance slit of a monochromator is both higher and wider than the source dimensions and the input optics serve to fill this area with light, thus ensuring that much more energy enters the monochromator than could be obtained with the source at the entrance slit.

3.4.1.2 Power output from a monochromator. For a radiation source emitting a continuous spectrum, Johns and Rauth (1965) have shown that the radiant flux $\phi(\lambda)$ centred at wavelength λ at the exit slit of a grating monochromator having equal entrance and exit slit widths, is given by the expression

$$\phi(\lambda) = L_s(\lambda)\,(\Delta\lambda)^2\,D_\theta(h_1/f_t)\,(W_g h_g \cos\theta)\,(\eta_c\eta_g\eta_t)\ \mathrm{W}, \tag{3.5}$$

where $L_s(\lambda)$ is the spectral radiance of the source image at the entrance slit in $\mathrm{W\,m^{-2}\,sr^{-1}\,nm^{-1}}$ at wavelength λ. Ideally $L_s(\lambda)$ should be equal to the brightness of the source itself at wavelength λ, but in practice it will be less than this because of losses in the input optics. $\Delta\lambda$ is the bandwidth of the monochromator defined as

$$\Delta\lambda = W_2/(f_t D_\theta)\ \mathrm{nm}, \tag{3.6}$$

where W_2 is the width of the exit slit, f_t is the focal length of the telescope mirror and D_θ is the angular dispersion ($\mathrm{rad\,nm^{-1}}$) of the diffraction grating. In general, monochromators designed for clinical use employ collimator and telescope mirrors with the same focal length, and entrance and exit slits of equal width (W_1 and W_2 respectively) and height (h_1 and h_2 respectively). The term $W_g h_g \cos\theta$ represents the projected area of the grating perpendicular to rays of wavelength λ from the collimating mirror, where W_g and h_g are the width and height of the grating respectively and θ is the angle between the plane of the grating and the parallel bundle of rays of wavelength λ from the collimating mirror. Finally the terms η_c, η_g and η_t represent the fraction of radiation of wavelength λ

reflected at the collimating mirror, grating and telescope mirror respectively.

Examination of equation (3.5) will show that the output power is directly related to the following:

(a) the radiance of the source;

(b) the square of the bandwidth—four times the power output can be achieved if twice the bandwidth is acceptable;

(c) the angular dispersion of the grating—a grating with twice the number of lines per mm (and hence twice the angular dispersion) should give twice the output;

(d) the angle subtended by the entrance slit at the centre of the collimating mirror (h_1/f_t); and

(e) the efficiency of the optical components of the whole instrument.

3.4.1.3 Spectral profile at the exit slit. The intensity distribution of wavelengths emerging from the exit slit of the monochromator will depend upon the entrance slit width, W_1, and the exit slit width, W_2.

When $W_1 \ll W_2$, a distribution of wavelengths from $\lambda - \Delta\lambda/2$ to $\lambda + \Delta\lambda/2$ appears at the exit slit, the intensity across the exit slit having the same shape as $L_s(\lambda)$, which for small slit widths can be approximated as flat, as illustrated in figure 3.7(*a*) $\Delta\lambda$ is given by equation (3.6).

When $W_1 = W_2/2$, the spectral profile is trapezoidal in shape [*see* figure 3.7(*b*)], the wavelengths present extending from $\lambda - 3\Delta\lambda/4$ to $\lambda + 3\Delta\lambda/4$. Finally, for the usual case of $W_1 = W_2$, a triangular distribution is obtained as shown in figure 3.7(*c*), the width of the distribution at half the peak intensity being equal to $\Delta\lambda$. The total wavelength range at the exit slit for any combination of entrance and exit slit widths is given by

$$\Delta\lambda_{\text{total}} = (W_1 + W_2)/(f_t D_\theta)\ \text{nm}. \tag{3.7}$$

However, in practice the pass band is greater than these ideal values given above due to aberrations in the optical components and the presence of stray radiation at remote wavelengths.

3.4.1.4 Dispersion element. Clinical irradiation monochromators have been constructed and used in which the dispersion element has been either a quartz enclosed water prism (e.g. Magnus *et al* 1959) or a blazed, ruled diffraction grating (e.g. Mackenzie and Frain-Bell 1973). A blazed grating has the advantage over a symmetrical, ruled reflection grating in that it concentrates 60–70% of the incident energy into just one of the spectral orders, with only a small amount of energy in the other orders.

In general the blazed ruled diffracton grating is preferred to the water prism as the dispersion element for use in the ultraviolet for the following two reasons:

(a) the dispersion is independent of wavelength; and

(b) it produces less spectral impurity, or stray radiation, to contaminate the exit beam.

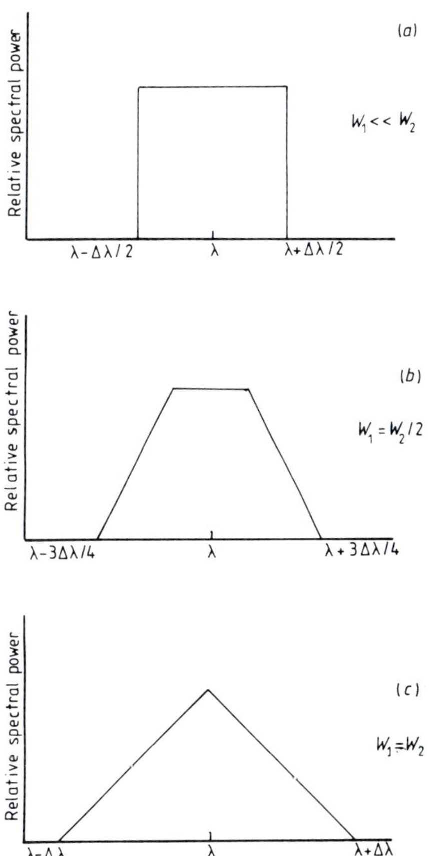

Figure 3.7 The effect of the entrance slit width W_1, and the exit slit width W_2 on the bandwidth $\Delta\lambda$ and spectral distribution at the exit slit of a monochromator.

Any radiation observed between the main diffracted orders in excess of that predicted by Fraunhofer diffraction is regarded as spectral impurity. In general there are four types of unwanted radiation, in addition to Fraunhofer diffraction, that can arise in the spectrum. These are known as ghosts, satellites, grass and diffuse scatter (Palmer *et al* 1975) and arise from imperfections in the machinery used to make the gratings. The largest requirement for ruled diffraction gratings, in terms of numbers, is for small replicas with areas in the range 25×25–$50 \times 50\ mm^2$. The most common type is a 1200 lines mm^{-1} grating blazed for 300 or 500 nm. The tolerances are quite modest, for example, 50% of the theoretical resolution, and ghosts $<10^{-4}$ of the main order intensity.

In more recent years holographic, or interference, gratings have become available. The feature of the interference technique used in the manufacture of these gratings is that there are no short-term errors in groove position and so the gratings generate no ghosts or grass, which results in a stray radiation level of one to two orders of magnitude lower than a contemporary ruled grating.

3.4.2 Monochromator performance

Clinical photosensitivity testing with an irradiation monochromator tends to be a time consuming investigation, particularly if the patient is to be irradiated with a range of doses at several different wavelengths. Because of this it is important to ensure that the system is operating near or at its optimum efficiency so as to minimise the strain on the patient of remaining still for lengthy periods of time and consequently to obtain more reliable results.

The power emerging from the exit slit of a monochromator is dependent upon several factors, as may be seen from equation (3.5). Some of the terms in this equation, notably h_1/f_t and $W_g h_g \cos\theta$, are features of the particular manufacturing design and are outside the influence of an investigator who merely wishes to purchase an 'off-the-shelf' system and not become involved in optical engineering.

The bandwidth selected, $\Delta\lambda$, will obviously have an important effect on output and the chocie of $\Delta\lambda$ in any situation will reflect the reasons for wishing to investigate the patient with a monochromator.

However, there still remain several terms in equation (3.5) which will affect the output, and the responsibility to ensure that these variables are maximised rests with the user.

Firstly, it is important that an image of the arc is efficiently focused onto the entrance slit and that the collimating mirror is filled with light. The position of the arc and the input optics with respect to the entrance slit will affect not only the monochromator output but also the spatial uniformity of radiation at the exit slit. Most irradiation monochromators incorporate mechanisms for vertical and lateral adjustment of the arc source, together with focusing adjustment of the condensing lens. The system can be set up roughly by setting the monochromator to pass green light, say, and holding a piece of white card at the exit slit. The lamp and condensing lens are adjusted until the most spatially uniform, intense image, as judged by eye, is obtained at the exit slit. Fine tuning can then be carried out by placing a detector such as a thermopile at the exit slit and adjusting the lamp and lens for maximum output in the desired spectral region, since the focal length of the condensing lens will be a function of radiation wavelength.

The efficiency of a ruled grating is dependent not only on the angular dispersion D_θ, but also upon the 'blaze' wavelength of the grating. For ultraviolet photobiology it is customary to use a grating with a blaze angle appropriate for a wavelength of 300 nm. The grating will then operate most efficiently at 300 nm and at wavelengths nearby, but may not do so at remote wavelengths, such as 1000 nm, in which case it would be necessary to use another grating suited to this wavelength.

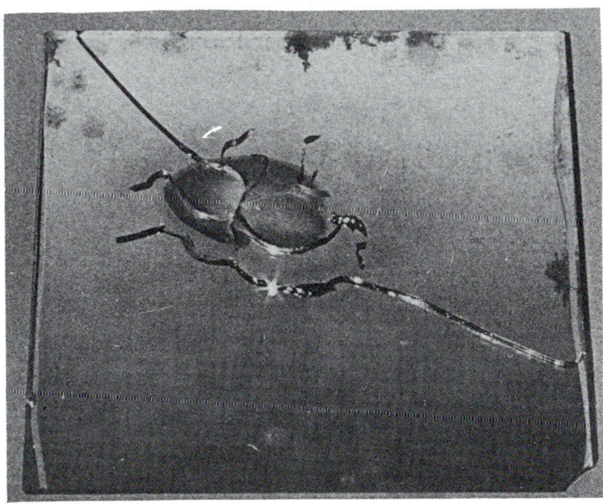

Figure 3.8 A plane mirror taken from a clinical irradiation monochromator. Note the deterioration of the surface where the entrance beam has impinged.

Finally the reflection of the radiation at each component will diminish as the optical surfaces of the mirrors and grating deteriorate due to the combined effect of heat, UVR and possibly ozone. Mirror surfaces should be inspected at intervals of say 200 h of usage. If the surfaces are contaminated with dust they should be cleaned with a mild liquid detergent and distilled water, care being taken not to leave small fragments of cotton wool, for example, on the surfaces after cleaning. Dirty mirrors will reflect diffusely and so give rise to stray radiation. If the surfaces still appear dull after cleaning they should be re-aluminised and preferably protected with a MgF_2 supercoat. A sure sign of optical surface deterioration is a more rapid fall-off in output of wavelengths less than about 320 nm compared to the visible. Figure 3.8 illustrates what can happen to a mirror in an irradiation monochromator if it is used well beyond its useful life.

Deterioration in the grating performance with use is difficult to check routinely.

3.4.3 Spectral impurity

The fraction of radiation emerging from the exit slit of a monochromator and outside the selected waveband is termed the 'spectral impurity' or more commonly, 'stray radiation'. The realisation that 100 times the energy is required for narrow band irradiation at 315 nm to produce a minimum skin erythema compared with that at 300 nm highlights the importance of spectral impurity. If an exposure dose of $2 \times 10^5\ J\,m^{-2}$ of radiation of wavelength 500 nm contained 0.1% of suburn radiation (UV-B and UV-C) as an impurity, the skin would receive a 'sunburn dose' of $200\ J\,m^{-2}$, which could be enough to cause a minimum erythema. The unsuspecting investigator might then erroneously believe that the patient is reacting abnormally to visible radiation.

The sectral impurity present at the exit slit is of two distinct types: firstly, stray radiation scattered towards the exit slit from inside the monochromator; and secondly, the second- or higher-order spectral radiation inherently produced by the diffraction grating. Stray radiation is produced by scattering and reflection from the internal structures and optical surfaces of the monochromator. This results in a background continuous spectrum of all wavelengths present at the entrance slit. The contribution of stray radiation to the total flux at the exit slit depends upon both the monochromator design and operation, and the conditions of the optical surfaces. Stray radiation may be reduced either by restricting the range of wavelengths entering the monochromator or by interposing suitable absorption filters between the exit slit and the specimen to be irradiated, e.g. the patient's skin.

Quantification of stray radiation is difficult, since there appears to be no generally accepted definition of this quantity nor a convention on how it should be measured and expressed. Also there are undoubtedly technical problems associated with its measurement. Stray radiation is highest in regions where the monochromator is set to pass wavelengths which are present in low relative intensities in the source spectrum. For xenon lamps this particularly applies to the UV-C region. A rough estimate of stray radiation can be made by using optical filters. For example, a photodetector with a flat spectral response is located at the exit slit and the monochromator is set to pass radiation of wavelength 260 nm with a bandwidth of 10 nm or less. The photodetector reading, R_1, is noted. A Schott colour glass absorption filter type WG305 is placed between the exit slit and the photodetector and the reading, R_2, noted. The ratio of unwanted to wanted radiation at the exit slit is then given approximately as $R_2/(0.915\ R_1 - R_2):1$. The factor 0.915 accounts for reflection losses at the air–filter interface (*see* §3.3.3.1). Spectral information on stray radiation can only be achieved by using a spectroradiometer of known stable characteristics carefully coupled to the output of the monochromator and incorporating a detector of known spectral sensitivity capable of handling a very wide range of radiation levels.

For single dispersion device monochromators used with xenon arc lamps the stray radiation due to wavelengths shorter than the wavelength of interest should not constitute more than 1% of the energy output at that wavelength. However, when the monochromator is set to pass wavelengths less than 300 nm the presence of long-wave UVR and visible radiation may constitute a significant fraction of the output power, and eventually of course the stray radiation will rise to 100% of the output when the wavelength dial is set below the cut-off wavelength of the lamp envelope.

3.4.4 Routine measurements associated with clinical irradiation monochromators

In order that scientifically meaningful and clinically useful results be obtained after testing a patient with an irradiation monochromator, it is important that the characteristics of the radiation beam incident upon the patient have been measured and well understood. From this point of view the physicist has a useful role to play in collaborating with the dermatologist or photobiologist wishing to study the behaviour of normal or abnormal skin with radiation of different wavelengths.

The measurements that can usefully be carried out include estimation of the output irradiance over the required range of wavelengths, checking the wavelength calibration of the monochromator, measuring the bandwidth of the radiation beam at the exit slit, measuring the spatial uniformity of the exit beam, and possibly estimating the magnitude of stray radiation.

3.4.4.1 Output irradiance. The output irradiance should be measured under the conditions in which it is proposed to irradiate the patient. The detector employed should preferably be a wavelength independent detector such as the Hilger Schwarz thermopile, type FT17 (Rank Hilger) which incorporates a silica window and sensitive element of 2 mm in

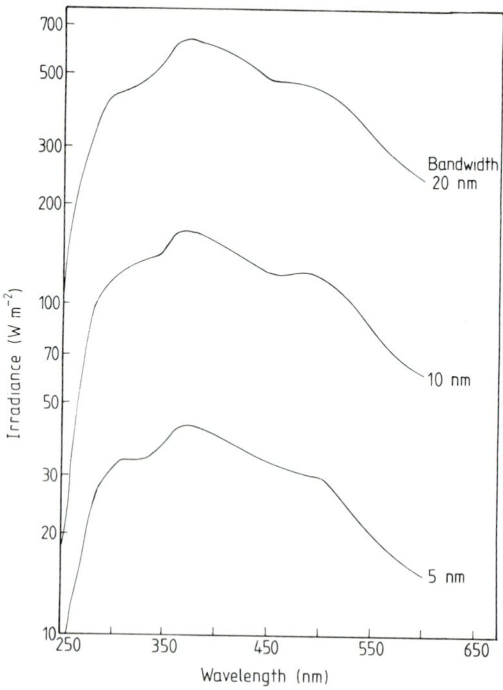

Figure 3.9 Output irradiance from a single grating monochromator used in conjuction with a 900 W xenon compact are lamp for an exit beam area of 10 × 10 mm^2.

diameter (*see* § 4.3.1). It is important that whatever detector is used the dimensions of the sensitive element should be less than the dimensions of the radiation beam. Figure 3.9 illustrates the measured output irradiance for bandwidths of 5, 10 and 20 nm and for an image size of $10 \times 10\ \text{mm}^2$ from a single grating instrument used in conjunction with a 900 W xenon compact arc source (Applied Photophysics Ltd.). This instrument incorporates a plane reflection grating with an area of $50 \times 50\ \text{mm}^2$, blazed at 300 nm and ruled at 1200 lines mm^{-1} giving disperson of 4 nm mm^{-1}. The entrance and exit slit heights are set by the manufacturer at 21 mm but the slit widths are fully adjustable from 0 to 8 mm corresponding to bandwidths of up to 32 nm. The light from the arc source is focused by an adjustable quartz lens doublet onto the entrance slit, a dynamic water cell being placed between the lens and the entrance slit to act as a heat filter. The complete instrument, shown in figure 3.10, has been used by the author both to irradiate human skin and also to study the optical properties of polymer films used as UVR dosimeters (*see* Chapter 7).

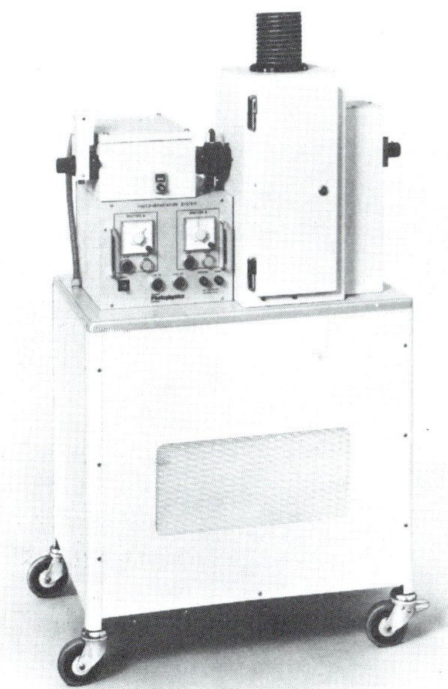

Figure 3.10 An irradiation monochromator (Applied Photophysics Ltd, London, UK).

3.4.4.2 Wavelength calibration. Most clinical irradiation monochromators incorporate a xenon lamp as the source of radiation principally because it exhibits a continuous spectrum which extends down to wavelengths below 250 nm (depending upon the lamp envelope material). However the spectrum from such a lamp exhibits no prominent lines in the UV or visible (*see* figure 2.13) and for this reason it is not readily suitable for use in calibrating the wavelength dial setting of the monochromator. Instead this can be achieved by employing a source which emits a line spectrum with neglible associated continuum such as a low-pressure mercury vapour lamp (*see* figure 2.6). The radiation from this source is focused onto the entrance slit, the entrance and exit slits adjusted to give a bandwidth of about 1 nm and the wavelength dial set to 546 nm. Under these conditions a green image should be observed at the exit slit. If this is not the case, the wavelength dial should be adjusted, i.e. the dispersion device rotated, until the mercury green line is observed at maximum brightness. The wavelength calibration of the monochromator can then be set by removing the wavelength dial, taking extreme care not to rotate the grating (or prism), setting the dial to correspond to 546 nm, and refitting the dial. If this procedure is carried out carefully, the wavelength dial can be turned to 436 nm and the mercury blue line will be observed.

3.4.4.3 Bandwidth determination. Once the wavelength dial has been properly adjusted using the low-pressure mercury vapour lamp, the same source can be used to determine the bandwidth for a variety of slit widths. This can be achieved as follows. A photodetector is located at the exit slit and the reading, R, recorded when the wavelength dial is set at 546 nm. The wavelength is slowly decreased until the photodetector reads $R/2$. This wavelength, λ_1, is noted. The wavelength is then increased beyond 546 nm until the photodetector again reads $R/2$ at some wavelength λ_2. The bandwidth $\Delta\lambda$ is then given by

$$\Delta\lambda = \lambda_2 - \lambda_1. \tag{3.8}$$

It should be remembered that if the dispersion device is a prism, the bandwidth will be a function of wavelength and so should be determined over the range of wavelengths of interest.

Knowledge of the bandwidth is particularly important if some biological effect is to be studied in a wavelength region in which the effect varies rapidly with wavelength. The classical example is the determination of the minimal erythema dose (MED) in human skin at different wavelengths. By combining the spectral distribution of radiation at the exit slit, which is principally a function of slit width, with the erythema action spectrum (*see* figure 5.4), it is possible to calculate the radiant exposure (dose) required to produce an MED as a function of bandwidth. The results of a series of such calculations at various central wavelengths show that at wavelengths near the peak of the action spectrum (around 295 nm), the dose required to produce an MED increases significantly with increase in bandwidth. Conversely wavelengths which are apparently ineffective at narrow bandwidths, i.e. $\lambda > 315$ nm will produce erythema if the bandwidth is sufficiently wide. This phenomenon should be borne in mind when carrying out determinations of MED's and comparing the results with those of other workers.

3.4.4.4 Spatial uniformity of exit beam. In clinical irradiation monochromators it is often customary to incorporate exit optics, for example a cylindrical lens or mirror, at the exit slit to produce a more acceptable beam cross section for patient irradiation. However it is important to bear in mind two conflicting aspects of beam size. Firstly, the study of action spectra in the various dermatoses often necessitates irradiation of multiple skin sites which may be as many as 100 or more in the one patient, so that the smaller the individual site is, the better. On the other hand, in small areas of skin it is often difficult to recognise abnormal morphological changes other than simple erythema. Considering both these factors an irradiation field of between 5×5 mm^2 and 10×10 mm^2 is normally employed. Having decided upon an irradiation field size, optimum uniformity of irradiance within this field can be achieved by adjustments to the entrance optics and the arc position (*see* § 3.4.2). If the field appear visually uniform, then measurements of irradiance within the field using a detector whose sensitive element is much smaller than the field (e.g. the Hilger Schwarz FT17 thermopile) should suggest that the irradiance is uniform to within $\pm 10\%$.

4 Ultraviolet Radiation Dosimetry

The physicist needs no persuasion as to the importance of the measurement of radiation. The correlation of data obtained by different workers, the avoidance of accidental over or under exposure of the patient, the study of the physiological effects produced by equal amounts of energy at different wavelengths, and the interpretation of clinical results, all demand precise quantitative data. Experience has shown that careful measurement leads to a better understanding of the biological mechanisms at work and ultimately to improved diagnosis and treatment for the patient.

The ultraviolet radiation produced by all the incoherent sources (non-laser) used in medicine and photobiology is not monochromatic, but consists of either a number of monochromatic lines (e.g. the Kromayer lamp, *see* § 2.3.3.3), or else has a continuous spectral distribution with perhaps some lines superimposed (e.g. UV-A fluorescent lamp, *see* § 2.3.2.5). In order to describe the radiation emitted by the lamp completely, it is necessary to give the distribution of energy as a function of wavelength. However in many situations where the interest lies in some particular action of the UVR, the effectiveness of the radiation is obtained by weighting the spectral distribution according to the appropriate function of wavelength and then integrating over all wavelengths for which the spectral content of the source is non-zero. (This summation assumes that the actions of the separate spectral components are independent and combine in a simple additive manner, that is, no synergistic or protective interactions exist between wavelengths.) The determination of this single quantity, the biologically effective irradiance, is most often the goal of clinical ultraviolet dosimetry, and may be achieved either by measuring the spectral distribution and then calculating the integral, or by direct measurement using a radiation detector whose sensitivity varies with wavelength according to the prescribed weighting function.

This chapter will address itself primarily to this problem. The terms and units appropriate to UVR dosimetry will be defined, followed by a description of the optical performance of some radiation detectors, and finally by a discussion of the techniques for carrying out clinically relevant measurements.

4.1 Radiometric Terms and Units

In clinical and photobiological UVR dosimetry it is customary to use the terminology of radiometry rather than that of photometry, since photometry is based on visible light measurements that simulate the human eye's photopic response curve and, strictly speaking, a source that emits only UVR has a zero-intensity in photometric terms.

The common radiometric terminology is listed in table 4.1. Terms relating to a beam of radiation passing through space are the 'radiant energy' and 'radiant flux'. Terms relating to a source of radiation are the 'radiant intensity' and the 'radiance'. The term 'irradiance', which is the most commonly used term in photobiology, relates to the object (e.g. patient) struck by the radiation. The radiometric quantities in table 4.1 may also be expressed in terms of wavelength by adding the prefix 'spectral'.

Table 4.1 Radiometric terms and units.

Term	Unit	Symbol	Definition
Wavelength	nm	λ	
Radiant energy	J	Q	
Radiant flux	W	ϕ	dQ/dt
Radiant intensity	$W\,sr^{-1}$	I	$d\phi/d\Omega$
Radiance	$W\,m^{-2}\,sr^{-1}$	L	$d\phi/d\Omega dA\cos\theta$
Irradiance	$W\,m^{-2}$	E	$d\phi/dA$
Radiant exposure	$J\,m^{-2}$	H	$E\cdot t$

The time integral of the irradiance is strictly termed the 'radiant exposure', but is sometimes expressed as 'exposure dose', or even more loosely as 'dose'. The term 'dose' in photobiology is analogous to the term 'exposure' in radiobiology and not to 'absorbed dose'. As yet the problems of estimating the energy absorbed by the critical target in the skin (whatever that might be) remain unsolved.

4.2 The Measurement of Ultraviolet Radiation

Techniques for the measurement of UVR may be divided into three classes: physical, chemical and biological. In general physical devices measure power, whilst chemical and biological systems measure energy.

The use of chemical methods, which measure the chemical change produced by the radiation, is called actinometry. These techniques have a place in photobiological studies dealing with microbiological specimens, but a description of the methods is out of context here.

Biological techniques of measurement are generally limited to the use of viruses and micro-organisms. The human skin has been used, and still is used in physiotherapy, as a UVR dosimeter in an indirect fashion; treatment times are determined by exposing small areas of the patient's skin to increasing exposures from a UV lamp and noting that exposure which produces a given degree of erythema (reddening of the skin, or sunburn).

4.3 Physical UVR Detectors

Ultraviolet radiation detectors consist of two basic physical types: thermal and photon. Thermal detectors respond to heat or power and have a uniform response over the spectral region for which the absorbance is near unity. The two examples of thermal detectors discussed in this section are the thermopile, which is based on the thermoelectric effect, and the relatively new pyroelectric detector which is based on the change in polarisation of a crystal when it undergoes a variation in temperature.

Photon detectors operate on the principle of the liberation of charge carriers by the absorption of a single quantum of radiation. Photon detectors, consequently, tend to have a non-linear spectral response. Examples of photon detectors which are covered here include the vacuum photodiode and photomultiplier, which rely on the photoelectric effect, and solid state photodiodes, which are based on the production of electron–hole pairs in a semiconductor.

4.3.1 Thermopiles

The most fundamental physical instrument for measuring radiant power is the thermopile which, for many years, has provided the basis for calibrating all other types of UV measurement systems. The principle of operation of the thermopile is based on the Seebeck or thermoelectric effect, whereby an EMF is generated when heat is applied to the junction of two dissimilar metals.

A schematic diagram of the Schwarz thermopile is shown in figure 4.1. Radiation transmitted through the window is absorbed by the receiving element (usually gold or platinum) which is blackened for maximum absorption. Two cone-shaped semiconductors (one p-type and one n-type) are spot welded to its underside to form the 'hot' junction. The 'cold' junction is between the semiconductors and their platinum electrodes embedded in a metal block of high thermal capacity. The components are housed in a glass envelope which may be evacuated for increased sensitivity. A window is inset into one end of the envelope to allow radiation to fall onto the receiving element. The choice of window material is governed by the spectral region of interest; for the UV, fused silica is most commonly used as this has a high, uniform transmission of radiation from 250–2200 nm.

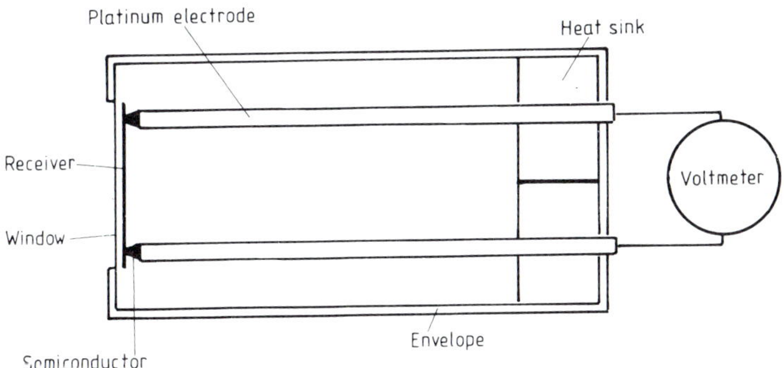

Figure 4.1 A schematic diagram of a thermopile. (Courtesy of Rank Hilger, Margate, England.)

In medical photobiology the Hilger Schwarz FT17 vacuum thermopile has been employed to measure the irradiance due to collimated beams of radiation, for example, the output from an irradiation monochromator (*see* §3.4.4.1). This device incorporates a circular receiving element of 2 mm in diameter together with a compensated element of similar dimensions which is screened from the direct radiation. The two elements are connected in opposition in order to minimise drift which can arise from variations in ambient temperature. The sensitivity of the FT17 thermopile is ~20 $W\,m^{-2}\,mV^{-1}$. More recently a wide-angle thermopile

(Rank Hilger FT32) has been developed which can be used to measure irradiance from extended, linear sources of UVR. A photograph of this device is shown in figure 4.2.

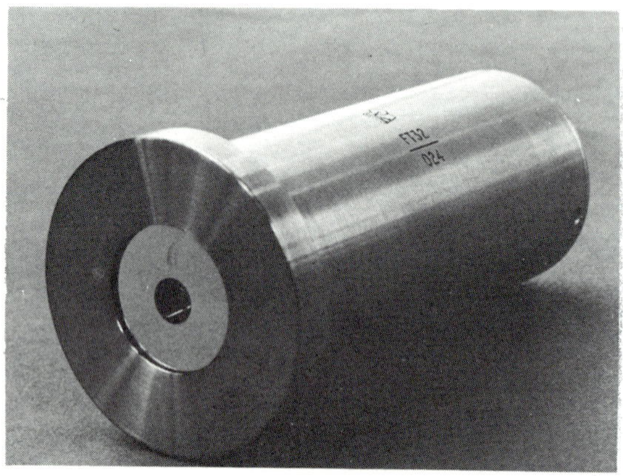

Figure 4.2 The FT32 wide-angle thermopile. (Courtesy of Rank Hilger, Margate, England.)

The thermopile is a valuable tool for the absolute determination of irradiance. However it is fragile and expensive and is not ideally suited for use as a routine instrument in the clinical environment. Its main role in the medical physics department is as a calibration instrument for more robust UV measuring devices. The thermopile can be calibrated at national standardising laboratories. The UK National Physical Laboratory calibrates thermopiles by comparing their response to the radiation from a tungsten filament lamp at a colour temperature of 2850 K with a standard thermopile. The responsivity determined in this manner has a stated uncertainty of the order of 1% at an irradiance of around $10\ \mathrm{W\,m^{-2}}$.

4.3.1.1 Theory of thermopile operation. The thermopile is basically a heat engine which converts heat energy into electrical energy. The thermal efficiency η of a heat engine is defined as

$$\eta = \Delta\theta/\theta_h, \tag{4.1}$$

where $\Delta\theta$ is the temperature difference between the hot and cold junctions and θ_h is the absolute temperature of the hot junction. In a typical thermopile $\Delta\theta$ is usually <1 K and may be as low as 10^{-6} K, whilst θ_h is of the order of room temperature. The generated EMF is related to $\Delta\theta$ by

$$\text{EMF} = \Delta\theta(P_p + P_n), \tag{4.2}$$

where P_p and P_n are the thermoelectric powers of the p-type and n-type semiconductors respectively.

In order to optimise the efficiency, and hence the generated EMF, the heat losses must be kept low so that $\Delta\theta$ is maximised.

Four types of heat loss occur in a thermopile; convection; re-radiation; conduction; and the Peltier effect (current produced by thermopile acts to reduce $\Delta\theta$). Convection losses depend upon the nature of the gas and the dimensions of the receiver and elements. These losses can be eliminated by evacuating the glass envelope which houses the components. Radiative losses from the hotter receiver and elements to the colder surroundings depend upon the temperature and emissivity of the surfaces involved. Radiative losses are unavoidable but can be minimised by making the back of the receiver highly reflecting. The most important loss is by conduction of heat through the elements from the hot to the cold junction. The losses due to the Peltier effect are negligible.

If the convection and Peltier losses are neglected, then $\Delta\theta$ can be expressed as

$$\Delta\theta = \varepsilon A/(L_r + L_c), \tag{4.3}$$

where ε is the energy absorbed in J m^{-2} s^{-1}; A is the area of the receiving element in m^2; and L_r and L_c are the heat losses in J K^{-1} s^{-1} due to radiative and conduction losses respectively.

Heat losses in the thermopile give rise to non-linearity in response. The Hilger-Schwarz FT17 thermopile has a published linear response up to an irradiance of 300 W m^{-2}, but at higher irradiances the measured irradiance can be appreciably less than the true irradiance. The thermopile should not be used at power levels above 2000 W m^{-2}, since the excessive heating of the sensitive element can cause permanent damage.

4.3.2 Pyroelectric detectors

Electrically calibrated pyroelectric radiometers (ECPR) are rapidly gaining acceptance as primary standards for the calibration of radiometric instruments, particularly in the United States. The sensor consists of a solid crystal that produces a change in current proportional to the rate of change of temperature of the crystal surface, which in turn is proportional to the rate of change of irradiance. The change in temperature alters the lattice spacings in the crystal which produces the change in electrical polarisation. Since no current is produced in the steady state it is necessary to modulate the incident radiation with an optical chopper. In order to maximise the changes in absorbed radiant energy, and hence temperature, the surface of the crystal is coated with a material such as gold black, which exhibits the following desirable properties: low reflectance (typically 0.5% in the visible); flat spectral response (±2% in the range 250–1600 nm); and relatively high thermal conductance compared to organic blacks. The active element in a typical sensor consists of a polished slab of lithium tantalate mounted on a thin plastic diaphragm. A thin-film resistive layer on the front surface serves as both a detector electrode and an electrical heater. The gold black optically absorbing layer is deposited on top of this.

The principle of operation of an ECPR is as follows. The incident radiation is chopped at a frequency of around 15 Hz with a 25% duty cycle. An electrical signal, 180° out of phase with the optical chopper, is generated and fed into the resistive heating element deposited onto the detector surface. This gives rise to a thermal signal in opposition to the chopped optical signal. The amplitude of the electrical signal is adjusted until a null is detected at the output of a synchronous rectifier. Under these conditions the optical power absorbed by the detector is nominally equal to the electrical drive power.

Absolute calibration of the ECPR—that is, determining the degree of equivalence between electrical and optical heating—is achieved by quantifying the following sources of variability and uncertainty: electrical calibration; reflectance and thermal resistance of the coating; spatial non-uniformity due to variations in detector thickness; heating in the leads to the heating element; and differences in the duty cycle for the chopped optical signal and generated electrical heating signal. Although these factors give rise to optical–electrical nonequivalence, their net effect is typically less than 1%.

A photograph of an ECPR suited for general radiometric use is shown in figure 4.3. This instrument is designed for use with three interchangeable pyroelectric sensors allowing measurement of irradiance in the range 10^{-4}–10^{6} W m^{-2}. The detectors have a flat spectral response with 99% of the incident radiation absorbed in the spectral range 400–3000 nm, dropping to 96% absorption in the range 250–16000 nm. The irradiance is stated to be accurate to ±1.5% of the reading.

The current price of a pyroelectric probe is comparable with that of

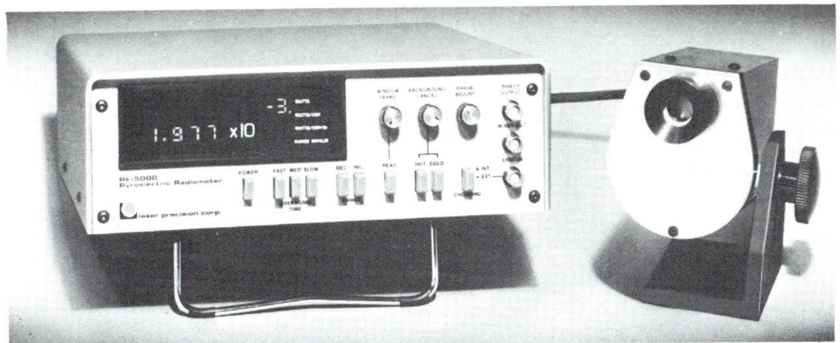

Figure 4.3 The Rk-5000 pyroelectric radiometer. (Courtesy of Laser Precision Corp, Irvine, California, USA.)

a thermopile (about £500), although the associated radiometer is about twice as expensive as the digital millivoltmeter required for use with a thermopile.

4.3.3 Phototubes

A phototube is basically a photoemissive cathode (photocathode) and a photoelectron collector (anode) housed in a vacuum or gas-filled envelope. A collection of various types of phototube is shown in figure 4.4

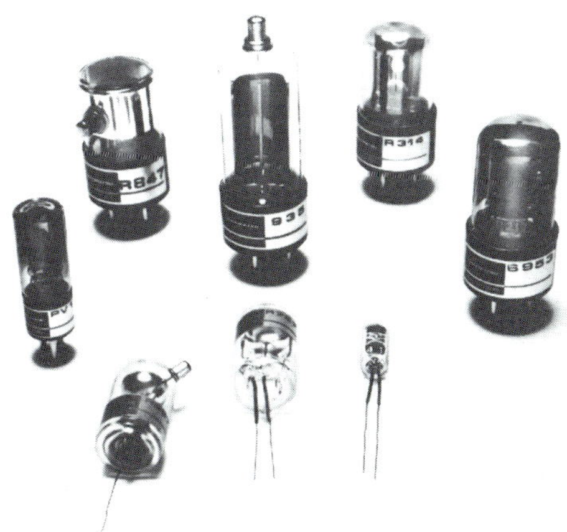

Figure 4.4 A collection of various phototubes. (Courtesy of Hamamatsu TV Co Ltd, Japan.)

The principle of operation of a phototube is based upon the photoelectric effect, whereby photons incident on the photocathode liberate electrons which are accelerated towards, and collected by, the anode. At a given wavelength of incident radiation the number of electrons emitted from the photocathode (tube current) is directly proportional to the number of photons striking the photocathode, resulting in a high degree of linearity over several orders of magnitude of intensity of incident radiation.

The spectral response of a phototube is determined by the photocathode material and the window material. A useful combination for a UV-C/UV-B detector is a phototube incorporating a Cs–Te photocathode with a fused silica window, which results in a phototube with a spectral response in the range 160–320 nm (so-called 'solar blind' device). The photocathode radiant sensitivities (in mA W^{-1}) of this and other common photocathode materials are shown in figure 4.5.

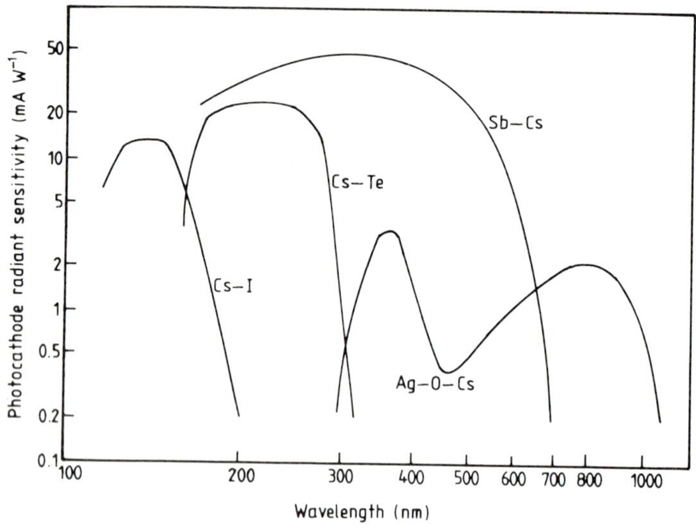

Figure 4.5 Some typical photocathode spectral response curves.

Vacuum phototubes are often the detectors of choice for portable ultraviolet radiometer systems. A vacuum phototube has been incorporated into an instrument (the IL730A UV actinic radiometer) which, with suitable filters and input optics, matches the wavelength response of the detector to the 'hazard action spectrum' for occupational exposure to UVR (*see* §7.4).

4.3.4 Photomultiplier tubes

A photomultiplier tube is essentially the same as a phototube, but with a built-in current amplifying section. The electron multiplier section consists of a chain of dynodes between the photocathode and anode. Electrons liberated at the photocathode are accelerated by a potential difference to the first dynode where they strike the dynode with sufficient kinetic energy to release additional electrons by the process of secondary emission. This process is repeated at each dynode such that the net effect is amplification of the primary photocurrent from the photocathode by a factor of 10^6 or more. The spectral response of photomultiplier tubes is governed by the same constraints applicable to phototubes.

The high internal amplification of photomultiplier tubes results in high sensitivity and low noise, and these detectors are ideal for use in instruments where a monochromator is used to isolate a narrow wavelength region and where consequently a low irradiance is generally incident upon the detector, e.g. in a spectroradiometer.

The disadvantages of photomultiplier tubes are their fragility and their requirement for a stable high-voltage power supply. Both these characteristics are drawbacks for a portable instrument.

4.3.5 Solid state photodiodes

In a solid state semiconductor with a reverse biased p–n junction (p material at a negative potential with respect to the n material), any free carriers which are generated are immediately swept by the electric field towards the region where there are majority carriers. If photons of sufficient energy are absorbed at or near the p–n junction, electrons will be excited from the valence band to the conduction band. The generation of excess electron–hole pairs across the junction gives rise to a current which can be measured in an external circuit. A p–n junction can be used therefore as a photoelectric detector, or photodiode. This mode of operation by applying a reverse bias across the junction is termed the 'photoconductive mode'.

Because of the internal potential rise in a p–n junction, photo-excited carriers are collected at the junction even in the absence of an external potential. If a resistor is placed across the terminals of the junction, a current passes through the resistor in proportion to the number of incident photons producing the potential difference across the p–n junction. This mode of operation of photodiodes is termed the 'photovoltaic mode'. This photovoltaic effect has widespread application in the familiar photographic exposure meter and in solar cell power supplies used on spacecraft, as well as in detectors for ultraviolet radiation.

Photodiodes are used in both the photoconductive and photovoltaic modes. In the photoconductive mode the device exhibits high sensitivity to incident radiation, but is prone to leakage currents resulting from changes in temperature. Temperature stability is better in the photovoltaic mode, but photosensitivity is lower.

A typical solid state photodiode is shown in figure 4.6. The device illustrated in this photograph is a Schottky-type GaAsP photodiode (type G1127). This detector has a photosensitive surface of 5 × 5 mm square mounted behind a fused silica window. It is suited for use in the UV, since its spectral response is in the range 180–680 nm.

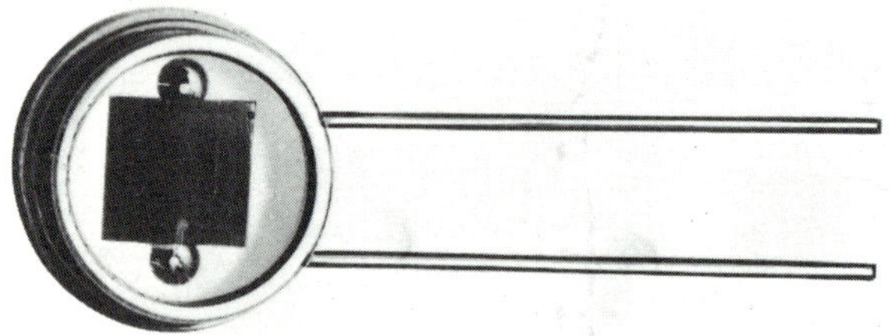

Figure 4.6 A GaAsP photodiode (type G1127). (Courtesy of Hamamatsu TV Co Ltd, Japan.)

The spectral response of solid state photodiodes depends upon the forbidden-energy gap of the semiconductor material. Materials which are used as photodiodes include silicon (Si), cadmium sulphide (CdS) and gallium arsenide phosphate (GaAsP). Silicon photodiodes have a peak spectral sensitivity in the near infrared and so their use for UV radiometry demands excellent rejection of longer wavelengths by filters or monochromators. Cadmium sulphide photodiodes also have a higher sensitivity in the visible and near infrared regions than in the UV. More recently GaAsP photodiodes have been developed which, unlike Si and CdS photodiodes, have no infrared response. A simple combination of such a photodiode with an ultraviolet transmitting colour glass filter (*see* figure 3.4) can result in a UV selective detector (e.g. the 'Uvichek' *see* figure 4.10). The spectral responses of typical Si and GaAsP photodiodes are compared in figure 4.7.

Solid state photodiodes are linear over a wide range of incident intensities (as much as ten orders of magnitude); have a response time which is usually better than 1 μs; and an operating temperature range of around −20 to +80°C.

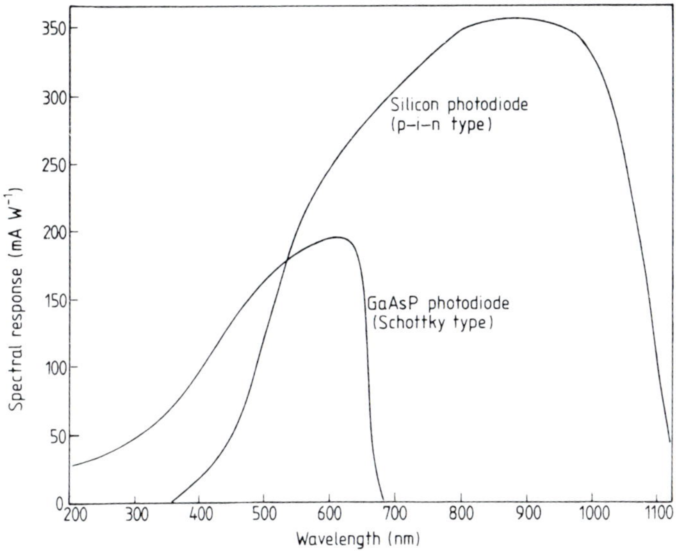

Figure 4.7 The spectral responses of a typical Si and of a typical GaAsP photodiode.

The low cost and small size of solid state photodiodes combined with their stability, robustness and simple electronic circuitry requirements, make them ideal detectors for portable instruments designed for use in the clinical environment.

4.4 Spectral Irradiance Measurements

In the introduction to this chapter the way in which a biologically effective irradiance could be determined, either by measuring the spectral irradiance at the point of interest and combining it with the effectiveness of the wavelengths present in the source for producing the required biological effect (action spectrum), or by using a detector whose spectral response matched the biological action spectrum, was explained. This section will discuss spectral irradiance measurements and in the next section the performance of detectors designed to measure a biologically effective irradiance directly will be examined.

In general, measurement of spectral irradiance can be achieved in two different ways: direct absolute measurement with a spectro-radiometer; or indirectly by combining the relative spectral power distribution of the source with an estimate of the total irradiance measured with a detector which has a flat spectral response over the wavelength range of the source, and a 180° field of view and a cosine-weighted response.

4.4.1 Direct measurement of spectral irradiance

A block diagram of the components required in a typical spectro-radiometer with data processing facilities is shown in figure 4.8.

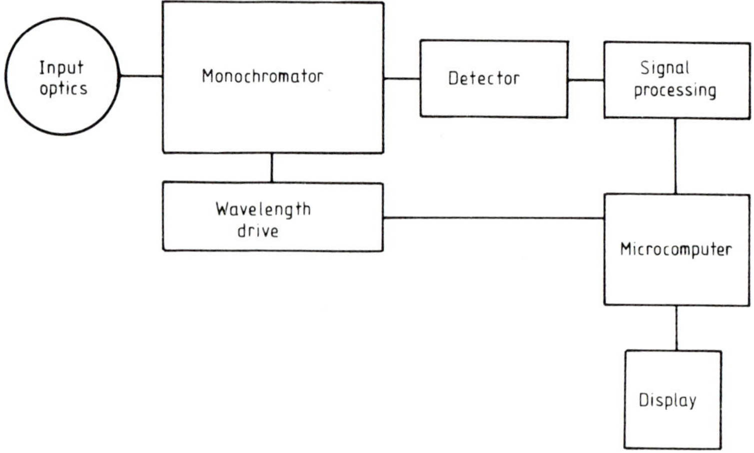

Figure 4.8 A schematic diagram of the principal components in a spectro-radiometer.

Radiation collected by the input optics passes through the entrance slit of the monochromator. A motor drives the wavelength drum of the monochromator at a constant speed. The analogue signal from the detector is integrated for a specified time interval and at the end of the interval the integrated signal is transferred to the computer and the cycle repeated. The wavelength drive and integrator output are synchronised such that the result of a spectral scan is a histogram of the source spectrum giving the irradiance in equal wavelength intervals throughout the spectrum.

The computer is not essential, but computer systems based on microprocessors are readily available nowadays and perform the useful functions of correcting the detector signal for the non-linear spectral response of the optical system, together with calculating the biologically effective irradiance, E_{BE}, according to

$$E_{BE} = \int E_s(\lambda)A(\lambda)\, d\lambda \text{ W m}^{-2}, \quad (4.4)$$

where the integration is over all wavelengths emitted by the source. $E_s(\lambda)$ is the spectral irradiance (W m^{-2} nm^{-1}) at wavelength λ nm, and $A(\lambda)$ is the relative effectiveness of radiation of wavelength λ in producing the desired biological effect, normalised to unity at some reference wavelength. The performance of the optical components of the spectro-radiometer will now be discussed.

4.4.1.1. Input optics. The spectro-radiometer should have a 180° field of view and a cosine-weighted angular response. This is particularly important for wide-area UV sources such as fluorescent lamps or sunlight. There are two types of input optics available for achieving these requirements. A roughly ground quartz hemispherical diffuser can be placed at the entrance slit of the monochromator, resulting in an approximate cosine response. Alternatively, an integrating sphere can be used, in which the radiation enters through a small aperature, with the entrance slit of the monochromator located at another aperture on the surface of the sphere. Because of multiple reflections within the sphere it is important that a diffuse coating with a high reflectance in the UV (e.g. MgO or Eastman 6080 $BaSO_4$ powder paint) be applied to the inside of the sphere to achieve good efficiency. Integrating spheres produce a cosine-weighted response, since the radiance through the entrance aperture varies as the cosine of the angle of incidence.

4.4.1.2 Monochromator. A ruled diffraction grating is normally preferred to a prism as the dispersion device in the monochromator used in a spectro-radiometer, mainly because of the independence of bandwidth with wavelength and better stray radiation characteristics. High performance spectro-radiometers, used for determining low-UV spectral irradiances in the presence of high irradiances at longer wavelengths, demand extremely low stray radiation levels. Such systems may incorporate a double monochromator—that is two single ruled grating monochromators in tandem—or, more recently, laser-holographically produced concave diffraction gratings can be used in a single monochromator.

4.4.1.3 Detector. Photomultiplier tubes, incorporating a photocathode with an appropriate spectral response, are normally the detectors of choice in spectro-radiometers. However if radiation intensity is not a problem, then solid state photodiodes may be used, since they require simpler and cheaper electronic circuitry.

4.4.1.4 Calibration and correction. The output signal $S(\lambda_0)$ from a spectro-radiometer set at wavelength λ_0 is related to the spectral irradiance incident on the receiving aperture of the instrument by the equation

$$S(\lambda_0) = \int_0^\infty E_s(\lambda)\, R(\lambda)\, \sigma\, (\lambda - \lambda_0)\, d\lambda, \tag{4.5}$$

where $E_s(\lambda)$ is the spectral irradiance at wavelength λ; $R(\lambda)$ is the spectral responsivity of the spectro-radiometer at wavelength λ; and σ is the slit function which is principally dependant on the entrance and exit slit widths of the monochromator (*see* § 3.4.1.3).

In many spectro-radiometric measurements the monochromator slit widths are sufficiently narrow that the slit function can be approximated by a delta function. Equation (4.5) then simplifies to

$$S(\lambda_0) = E_s(\lambda_0)\, R(\lambda_0). \tag{4.6}$$

The spectral responsivity is determined by measuring the spectro-radiometer's response to a source of known spectral irradiance. The standard source which is normally employed is a quartz-iodine lamp with a coiled tungsten filament operating at a colour temperature of about 3000 K. The spectral irradiance from the lamp is calibrated over the range 250–2500 nm by comparison with the radiance of a blackbody. Alternatively, deuterium lamps can be used as standard sources for calibration in the UV. The actual shape of the spectral responsivity function $R(\lambda)$ will depend upon many factors, such as the spectral efficiency of the diffraction grating and the photocathode material used in the detector. However it is not unusual for $R(\lambda)$ to decrease by a factor of ten from a wavelength of 350 nm to 250 nm, and so estimates of spectral irradiance in the UV, to even a moderate degree of accuracy, required prior knowledge of this function.

In high-precision spectro-radiometry, which may be required if the biologically effective irradiance is to be determined from a source whose spectrum is falling (e.g. sunlight, figure 2.1) in a wavelength region where the biological action spectrum is rising sharply (e.g. erythema action spectrum, figure 5.4), it may be necessary to take into account the slit function. To a first approximation the slit function of a monochromator with equal entrance and exit slit widths is a triangle (*see* figure 3.7). In reality, the slit function has broad wings which slowly approach zero after an initial rapid decrease of 3–7 orders of magnitude, depending on whether the monochromator has one or two dispersive elements. These wings mean that the spectro-radiometer can respond to radiant flux at wavelengths far removed from the wavelength setting λ_0 of the instrument. If the slit function $\sigma(\lambda - \lambda_0)$ is known it is possible to derive the spectral irradiance $E_s(\lambda_0)$ from the observed signal $S(\lambda_0)$ by deconvolution of equation (4.5).

4.4.2 Indirect measurement of spectral irradiance

Spectro-radiometers are expensive instruments and will not be available to the majority of hospital physicists. Nevertheless estimates of spectral irradiance may still be possible using less expensive instrumentation. The accuracy of indirect estimates of spectral irradiance will not be as high as achieved spectro-radiometrically, but may often be adequate for clinical purposes.

The total irradiance at the point of interest is simply equal to the integral of spectral irradiance over all wavelengths emitted by the source. The relative spectal intensity, or spectral power distribution, may therefore be reduced to absolute spectral irradiance by equating the integrated spectral power distribution to the total irradiance measured by a detector which has a uniform spectral response over the wavelength range of the source, and preferably a 180° field of view with a cosine-weighted response so that measurements can be performed on extended, linear sources. The spectral power distribution may be obtained either from the manufacturer's data or by means of a scanning monochromator and detector. It is not essential to incorporate input optics on the scanning monochromator since it is assumed that the spectral power distribution in the field of view of the entrance slit is representative of the spectral irradiance incident at the entrance slit. Although the response of the scanning monochromator/detector does not need to be absolutely determined, it is still important to estimate the spectral responsivity $R(\lambda)$ especially if measurements are to be carried out in a wavelength region where this function changes by a significant amount.

The author has measured the spectral irradiance from the lamps used in a whole body UV-A treatment cubicle using the following indirect technique.

The total irradiance, E, in $\mathrm{W\,m^{-2}}$, was measured at the point of interest using a FT32 thermopile (Rank Hilger). This device has a uniform wavelength response in the range 250–2200 nm, a wide field of view, and an approximately cosine-weighted angular response.

A Beckmann DBG spectrophotometer, modified to perform as a scanning monochromator, was used to determine the spectral power distribution from the UV-A lamps.

The analogue signal from the spectrophotometer was digitised by means of a voltage-to-frequency converter and the resultant pulses accumulated in a scalar. Every ten seconds the contents of the scalar were recorded on paper tape and the cycle repeated. During the 10 s data integration period, the wavelength change on the spectrophotometer was 1.70 nm. It was necessary to correct the recorded spectrum for the variation with wavelength of the sensitivity of the spectrophotometer. This was achieved by recording the spectrum of a 200 W quartz-iodine lamp of known spectral irradiance and deriving the spectral responsivity function $R(\lambda)$.

The photomultiplier tube employed in the Beckmann DBG Spectrophotometer was such that the efficiency of detection fell rapidly at wavelengths greater than about 650 nm. Since the thermopile will respond to wavelengths up to 2500 nm, it was necessary to make an estimate of the fraction of the measured irradiance in the near-infrared region. This was achieved by using a Schott red glass filter (type RG630), 3 mm thick and 50 mm in diameter. This filter transmits uniformly from 650 nm to beyond 2500 nm with 50% internal transmittance at 630 nm and negligible transmittance at wavelengths below 600 nm. Measurements with this filter indicated that 7% of the irradiance measured by the thermopile was due to wavelengths greater than 600 nm, and so the total irradiance, E, which is equated with the integrated spectral power distribution, needs to be reduced by this amount.

Hence the spectral irradiance in the wavelength interval $\lambda_i - \Delta\lambda/2$ to $\lambda_i + \Delta\lambda/2$ is given as

$$E_s(\lambda_i, \Delta\lambda) = (1 - 0.07)\, E\left[P(i)/\sum_{i=1}^{N} P(i)\,\Delta\lambda\right] \mathrm{W\,m^{-2}\,nm^{-1}}, \quad (4.7)$$

where λ_i is the central wavelength in the ith timing period; $\Delta\lambda$ is the wavelength increment during each data integration period ($\Delta\lambda$ =

1.70 nm); E is the total irradiance incident upon the detector; $P(i)$ is the number of pulses collected during the ith timing period corrected for nonlinearity of spectrophotometer response; and N is the number of timing periods ($N \sim 200$).

4.5. Biologically Weighted Irradiance Measurements

Probably the most common problem confronting the hospital physicist in clinical photobiology is the estimation of the biologically effective irradiance at the point of interest. Questions to be answered may include:

(1) How hazardous is this UV source?
(2) How effective is this lamp in producing erythema?
(3) What is the therapeutically effective radiance from this photochemotherapy treatment unit?

It has already been shown that the answers to these questions can be obtained by two different routes; measuring the spectral irradiance, or employing a detector whose spectral response matches the action spectrum of the appropriate biological effect. This section will discuss the latter method.

The instrumentation for directly assessing the exposure hazard from a UV source is described in §7.4 and will not be covered here. Instead we shall first consider the performance of UV-B ('erythema') detectors, followed by a discussion of UV-A ('photochemotherapy') detectors.

4.5.1 UV-B detectors

The best known acute biological effect in man following exposure to ultraviolet radiation is erythema. As is shown in figure 5.4, erythema is caused principally by wavelengths of less than 315 nm (UV-B and UV-C) and, since terrestrial sunlight, which is the most common environmental source of UVR, contains no UV-C, UV-B detectors are often synonomous with erythema monitors.

Clearly the only satisfactory UV-B detectors in this context are those whose spectral response closely matches the erythema action spectrum. By careful attention to optical engineering it is possible to produce a device which satisfies this criterion. However, many UV-B detectors have spectral responses which are significantly different from the erythema action spectrum and can lead to misleading estimates of the erythemal efficacy of a source if they are used injudicially, as is illustrated below.

One particular commercially-available model of a UV-B detector employs a GaAsP photodiode as the sensor, in conjunction with an optical filter which has a symmetrical wavelength response peaking at 310 nm with a bandwidth of 34 nm (*see* figure 4.9). The device is calibrated with monochromatic 310 nm radiation and so the meter reading in $\mathrm{W\,m^{-2}}$ only represents true irradiance for this one situation. For a UV source emitting any other spectral distribution, the meter reading will be dependent upon both the spectral irradiance and the spectral response of the detector. Nevertheless it is still possible to relate the meter reading to an erythemally effective irradiance by the relationship

$$\begin{matrix}\text{erythemally effective}\\ \text{irradiance (W m}^{-2}\text{)}\end{matrix} = \begin{matrix}\text{UV-B detector}\\ \text{reading (W m}^{-2}\text{)}\end{matrix} \cdot Q, \tag{4.8}$$

where Q is a correction factor which allows for the difference between the erythema action spectrum and the spectral response of the UV-B detector, and is given by

$$Q = \int P(\lambda)\,\varepsilon(\lambda)\,\mathrm{d}\lambda \Big/ \int P(\lambda)\,\nu(\lambda)\,\mathrm{d}\lambda, \tag{4.9}$$

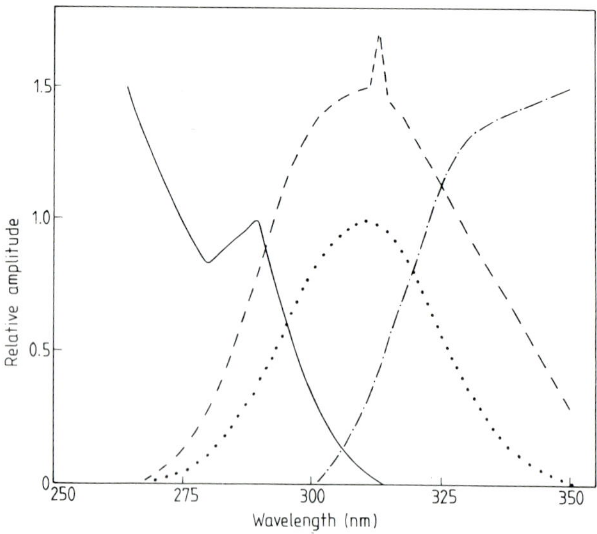

Figure 4.9 The spectral power distribution of a fluorescent sunlamp (broken curve) and of global UVR at a solar altitude of 60° and ozone layer thickness of 0.32 cm at STP (chain curve), together with the spectral response of a UV-B detector (dotted curve) and the erythema action spectrum for human skin (full curve).

where the integration is over all wavelengths emitted by the source. Here $P(\lambda)$ is the spectral power distribution (i.e. relative spectral intensity) at wavelength λ; $\varepsilon(\lambda)$ is the relative effectiveness of radiation of wavelength λ in producing erythema; and $\nu(\lambda)$ is the spectral response of the UV-B detector at wavelength λ, normalised to unity at 310 nm.

In the examples given below the erythema action spectrum which has been used is that published by Mackenzie and Frain-Bell (1973), normalised to unity at a wavelength of 290 nm (figure 4.9). This means that the erythemally effective irradiance given by equation (4.8) is that irradiance of monochromatic 290 nm radiation which would produce the same erythemal effect as the UV source in question. There is nothing especially significant about 290 nm as the reference wavelength, and indeed any wavelength can be chosen within reason. Note however that the numerical value of the erythemally effective irradiance will depend upon the reference wavelength.

Consider the result of using this UV-B detector to estimate the erythemally effective irradiance from a fluorescent sunlamp which has the spectral power distribution shown in figure 4.9. The value of the correction factor Q has been calculated to be 0.39. That is, the UV-B meter reading is overestimating the erythemally effective irradiance of the fluorescent sunlamp by a factor of 2.56. If now the detector is used to estimate the erythemal effectiveness of noontime summer sunshine in the UK (solar altitude 60°, ozone layer thickness equivalent to 0.32 cm at STP), as illustrated in figure 4.9, the correction factor is now only 0.011. The unsuspecting investigator, who naïvely equates the meter reading of a UV-B detector with erythemally effective irradiance, would overestimate this irradiance by a factor of 100! Clearly it cannot be emphasised too strongly that whenever UV-B detectors (or UV-C or UV-A, for that matter) are used to estimate the effective irradiance of some biological mechanism predominantly sensitive to that spectral region, due care and attention must be paid to the action spectrum of the biological effect, the spectral properties of the detector, and the spectral power distribution of the source.

4.5.2 UV-A detectors

Probably the most widespread use of ultraviolet radiation in clinical medicine nowadays is the treatment of the skin disease psoriasis by photochemotherapy (*see* §6.3). Basically, this treatment involves the administration of a photoactive drug followed a short while later by exposure of the patient to UV-A radiation in the type of treatment cubicle illustrated in figure 6.3. For successful treatment it is important to carry out regular monitoring of the UV-A irradiance at the patient surface. This has resulted in the availability of several different designs of UV-A detector. These devices generally incorporate a solid state photodiode, one or more optical filters, some simple electronic circuitry and a display. One such UV-A detector is shown in figure 4.10.

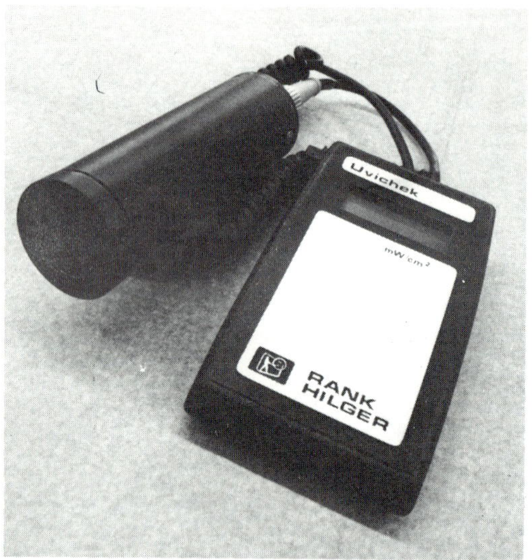

Figure 4.10 The 'Uvichek' UV-A detector. (Courtesy of Rank Hilger, Margate, England.)

The properties of the optical components used typically result in a spectral response from about 300–400 nm, peaking at around 360 nm, and an angular response which is often a poor approximation to a cosine-weighted response.

The spectral responses of three different models of UV-A detector commonly found in clinical practice are shown in figure 4.11. The curves have been normalised to unity at a wavelength of 365 nm for each UV-A detector. The fractional deviation of the angular response of each of these UV-A detectors from a cosine-weighted response is shown as a function of angle of incidence in figure 4.12. The fractional deviation at angle θ from the normal is defined as:

$$1 - \left(\frac{\text{meter reading at } \theta^\circ}{\text{meter reading at } 0^\circ} \Big/ \cos\theta\right). \qquad (4.10)$$

The meter reading in W m^{-2} generally refers to monochromatic irradiation at 365 nm incident normally on the sensor since calibration can be conveniently carried out using this strong mercury line. In fact, with a medium pressure mercury vapour lamp it is possible to isolate radiation at wavelengths between 350 nm and 380 nm, with over 96% of the radiation coming from the group of mercury emission lines between 365 nm and 367 nm. The considerations that applied to UV-B detectors for use with spectral power distributions other than the calibration wavelength, apply equally well to UV-A detectors. Indeed the radiation sources used in photochemotherapy treatment units are almost invariably UV-A fluorescent lamps with the spectral power distribution shown in figure 2.9.

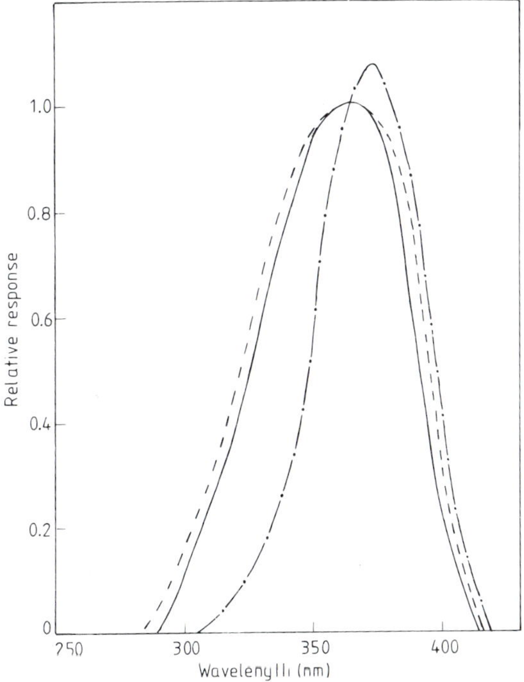

Figure 4.11 The spectral response of three commercially available UV-A detectors (after Stobbart and Diffey 1980): full curve, Uvichek (Rank Hilger, Margate, England); chain curve, PUVA Meter (Waldmann GmbH & Co, Villingen-Schwenningen, West Germany); and broken curve, Blak-Ray J221 (Ultraviolet Products Inc, San Gabriel, California, USA.)

The UV-A irradiance at a particular point exposed to the radiation from such a unit is simply equal to the integral of the spectral irradiance at that point over the UV-A range of wavelengths, that is, 315–400 nm. This may be expressed mathematically as:

$$\text{UV-A irradiance} = \int_{315}^{400} E_s(\lambda)\, d\lambda \ \mathrm{W\,m^{-2}}, \tag{4.11}$$

where $E_s(\lambda)$ is the spectral irradiance ($\mathrm{W\,m^{-2}\,nm^{-1}}$) at a wavelength λ nm.

If now a UV-A detector is placed at the point of interest, the meter

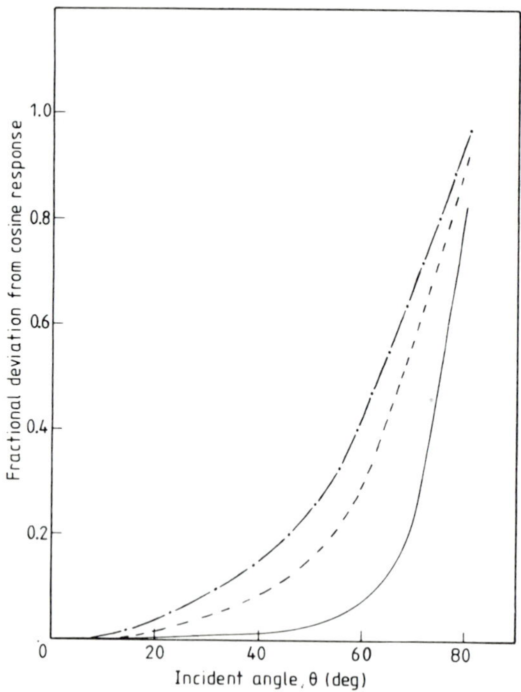

Figure 4.12 The angular response of three commercially available UV-A detectors (after Stobbart and Diffey 1980): full curve, Uvichek (Rank Hilger, Margate, England); chain curve, PUVA Meter (Waldmann GmbH & Co, Villingen-Schwenningen, West Germany); and broken curve, Blak-Ray J221 (Ultraviolet Products Inc, San Gabriel, California, USA.)

reading will be given by

$$\text{UV-A detector reading} = \int_A \int_\lambda E_s(\lambda)\, \nu(\lambda)\, G(A)\, d\lambda\, dA \ \text{W m}^{-2}, \quad (4.12)$$

where $G(A)$ is a complex geometrical function essentially related to the angular response of the UV-A detector. The integration is over A, the area of the lamp array. The spectral response of the detector at wavelength λ is given by $\nu(\lambda)$ and the integration is over all wavelengths for which the detector has a non-zero response. This means that unless the radiation source emits monochromatic radiation at 365 nm normally incident on the face of the sensor, the measured UV-A irradiance will differ from the true UV-A irradiance.

Ideally it is desirable to use a detector with a spectral response which matches the action spectrum for the regression of lesions in psoriasis. However, since this action spectrum still remains uncertain, perhaps the next best thing would be to use a detector which combined a cosine-weighted angular response with a flat spectral response from 315–400 nm and a zero response at all other wavelengths. This detector would measure true UV-A irradiance irrespective of the spectral power distribution of the source. Unfortunately such a detector does not exist for various physical reasons.

Nevertheless presently-used UV-A detectors can still enable computation of the true UV-A irradiance or even some biologial irradiance (assuming a therapeutic action spectrum is postulated) if there is access to the spectral power distribution of the radiation source, and the spectral response and angular response of the UV-A detector using a relationship analogous to equation (4.8).

5 The Biological Effects of Ultraviolet Radiation in Man

The observable biological effects in man due to exposure from external sources of ultraviolet radiation are limited to the skin and to the eyes because of the low penetrating properties of UVR in human tissues. This chapter will outline the optical properties and the recognisable short-term and long-term effects of UV exposure in the skin and the eyes.

5.1 Structure of the Skin

The skin consists of a superficial layer, the epidermis, and a deeper vascular connective tissue layer termed the dermis or corium. A schematic cross section of the superficial layers of the human skin perpendicular to the skin surface is given in figure 5.1.

The epidermis contains no blood or lymphatic vessels and is composed of stratified squamous epithelium which varies in thickness in different parts of the body. The superficial layer of the epidermis, termed the stratum corneum or horny layer, is a mechanically tough and chemically resistant layer. The epidermal cells are continually being manufactured by the keratinocytes (prickle cells) of the stratum malpighii. Keratinocytes are derived from a single germinative layer of basal cells. In normal skin it may take up to 14 days for a daughter cell of the basal layer to reach the stratum corneum and another one to two weeks before it is sloughed off from the skin surface. In the skin disease psoriasis the cell cycle is accelerated, the lifetime of a cell being reduced from about 28 days to something like 3 or 4 days. The increased number of skin cells and rapid cell kinetics that characterise the disorder lead to the formation of lesions that shed scales. There are specialised cells called melanocytes which reside within the basal layer and produce granules called melanosomes containing the pigment melanin. Melanin is a complex macro-

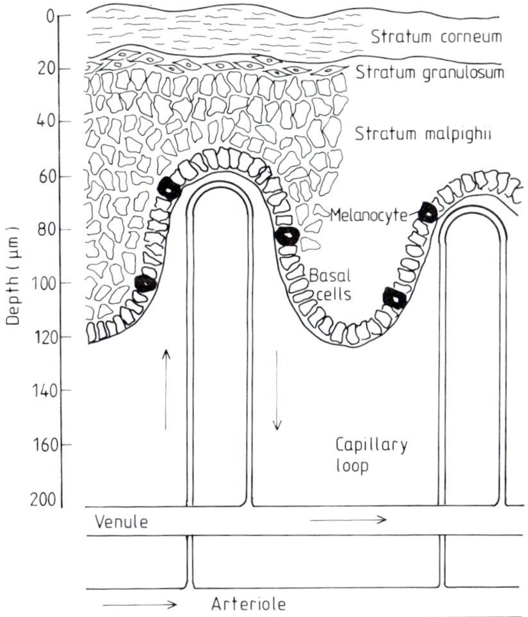

Figure 5.1 A schematic cross section of human skin perpendicular to the skin surface.

molecular protein which strongly absorbs light and UVR and plays an important role in protecting the viable cells against damage by UVR.

Below the epidermis lies the dermis, which has well-marked ridges and projections, called papillae, on its upper surface. This prevents a separation of the two layers by shearing. The dermis consists of dense connective tissue with blood vessels and lymphatics, and merges into the less dense subcutaneous tissue. It is the elastic fibres present in the dermis that give the skin its characteristic elasticity.

Finally, the skin over the entire body is supplied segmentally by nerves from the spinal cord. The nerve endings, or receptors, are responsible for cutaneous sensations such as touch, pain, heat and cold.

5.2 Optics of the Skin

Studies on the optics of the skin present severe experimental problems. The skin is not only reflecting and absorbing, it is inhomogeneous—

containing structures such as hair follicles, sweat glands and sebaceous glands—and even its dimensions are difficult to measure. Ultraviolet radiation incident on the skin may be reflected, refracted, absorbed, scattered, transmitted or produce fluorescence.

Early work on the penetration of visible and UV radiation in human skin was carried out by Bachem and Reed in 1930. These workers placed frozen sections of plantar skin over the slit of a spectrograph and determined the transmittance of the mercury lines through the stratum corneum, the viable layer of the epidermis and dermis. Their results are summarised in table 5.1, which gives the percentage of incident radiation transmitted though skin layers of defined thickness.

Table 5.1 Percentage transmission of visible and ultraviolet radiation at different depths in skin [Bachem and Reed (1930); adapted from Daniels (1969)].

Layer	Thickness of layer, mm	Wavelength, nm 200	250	280	300	400	550	750
Horny layer	0.03	0	19	15	34	80	87	78
+ Viable epidermis	0.05	0	11	9	16	57	77	65
+ Dermis	2.0	0	0	0	0	1	5	21

A comprehensive experimental study on the transmission through skin of visible and UV radiation was reported by Hansen in 1948. As a radiation source Hansen used a super high-pressure mercury arc lamp cooled by circulating distilled water. Spectral regions were separated with the help of optical fluid filters, solid filters or by a double monochromator, and dosimetry was carried out photographically. The results of the investigation showed that transmission of UVR through skin, both (depilated) mouse skin and human skin, and through frozen sections of different layers of both types of skin, decreases uniformly with wavelengths from 500–300 nm. In the study Hansen looked at the influence of scattering of UVR in the skin, reflection of UVR from the skin surface, fluorescence of the skin and width of the spectral interval. He concluded that the introduction of the various corrections needed did not alter the shape of the transmission curve, but only the numerical value of the transmission in the spectral region 280–500 nm. Apart from a minimum at 415 nm, due to absorption by the haemoglobin, the various layers of the skin did not exhibit any characteristic feature as regards the absorption of radiation.

The most recent study on the ultraviolet optics of human skin was carried out by Everett and his colleagues in 1966. These investigators treated both caucasian and negro skin in various ways to separate the stratum corneum and the entire epidermis. A recording spectrophotometer with integrating sphere input optics was used to measure the radiation absorbed, transmitted and scattered by each skin specimen. A comparison of the ultraviolet spectral transmission of specimens obtained with the different separation techniques showed them to be remarkably similar. Figure 5.2 shows the direct transmission and total transmission (direct plus scattered) for caucasian stratum corneum 10 μm in thickness. Note that of the 50% or so of incident UV-A transmitted through the stratum corneum to the viable cells of the epidermis, only about 5% is directly transmitted, the rest being scattered radiation. The direct and total transmission spectra for intact, whole epidermis, 26 μm in thickness, are compared in figure 5.3. As was observed for stratum corneum, the total transmitted radiation is appreciably greater than that directly transmitted by whole epidermis.

To date there have been few theoretical studies on the transport of UVR in skin, probably because of its complex nature. It may be possible

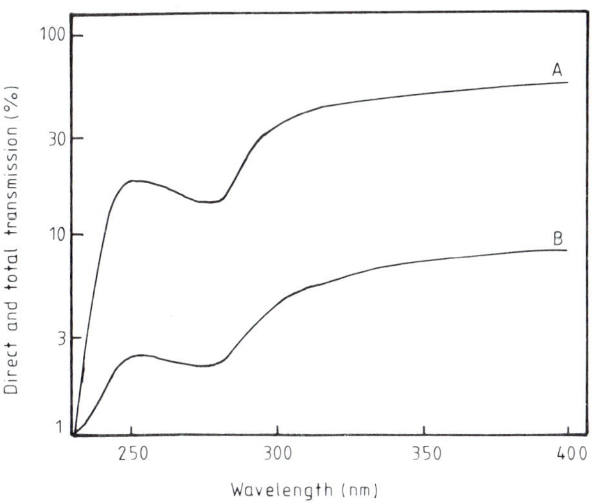

Figure 5.2 Direct (curve B) and total (curve A) transmission of ultraviolet radiation through Caucasian stratum corneum 10 μm in thickness (after Everett *et al* 1966).

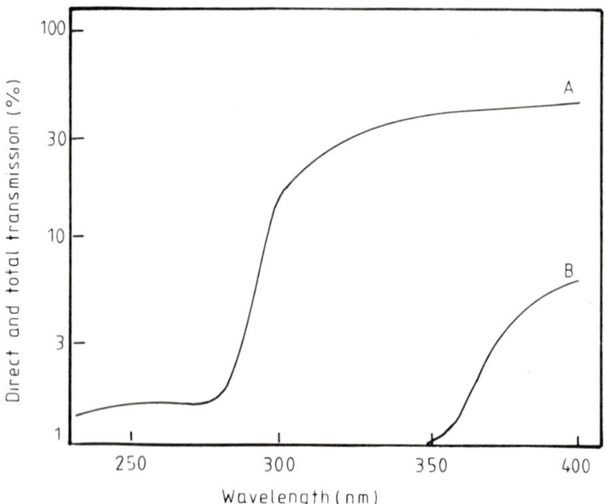

Figure 5.3 Direct (curve B) and total (curve A) tranmission of ultraviolet radiation through whole epidermis 26 μm in thickness (after Everett *et al* 1966).

that turbid medium theory, which is a particular case of the phenomenon of radiative transfer, could be applied to the theoretical study of skin optics. Turbid medium theories may be conveniently divided into two categories; those based upon continuum models and those based upon statistical models. However, many of the experimental data necessary to develop these models in skin are lacking.

5.3 Effects of Ultraviolet Radiation on Normal Skin

The normal responses of the skin to UVR can be classed under two headings: acute effects and chronic effects. An acute effect is one of rapid onset and generally of short duration, as opposed to a chronic effect which is often of gradual onset and long duration. These effects should be distinguished from acute and chronic exposure conditions which refer to the length of the UVR exposure. The acute reactions considered will be erythema (sunburn), delayed melanin pigmentation (suntan) and vitamin D production. Skin ageing and skin cancer will be discussed as those chronic reactions produced by prolonged or repeated UVR exposure.

5.3.1 Ultraviolet erythema

Exposure to UVR, particularly from wavelengths less than 315 nm, can result in erythema. The redness of the skin which is characteristic of erythema is attributable to an increased blood content by dilation of the superficial blood vessels, mainly the subpapillary venules. Sunburn caused by exposure to solar radiation normally has a latent period of a few hours. Erythema induced by artificial sources is strongly dependent on the wavelength of radiation. At 300 nm an average threshold dose or minimal erythema dose (MED) in unacclimatised white skin is about 200 $J\,m^{-2}$, whereas for UV-A radiation the MED is about a thousand-fold higher. Larger doses of UV-B may result in oedema, pain and blistering, although blistering seldom occurs with UV-C.

5.3.1.1 The mechanism of ultraviolet erythema. The vascular response due to UVR could be considered to arise from two different types of mechanism. It could be from a direct action on the vessel wall itself, or indirectly from a photochemical reaction via a diffusing chemical mediator arising in the epidermis. There is recent evidence that prostaglandins, a group of long-chain fatty acids with vasoactive properties, are implicated as possible mediators or modulators of inflammation in UV-C and UV-B erythema. It is observed that prostaglandin production increases following UVR exposure. However prostaglandins are thought not to play as important a role, if any, as mediators of the UV-A induced erythema, which may be due to a direct effect on dermal vasculature.

The evidence that UVR erythema entails diffusion of a chemical mediator from the epidermis to the dermis includes the following.

(1) The erythemally reactive UVR is mostly absorbed in the epidermis.

(2) There is a latent period between exposure and appearance of erythema.

(3) The phenomenon known as 'diffusion flush', which is that an erythema, elicited with a large dose of UVR, is after some time surrounded by a diffuse reddening, less intense than the central erythema and slowly spreading outward.

The diffusion theory of UVR erythema has been examined mathematically by van der Leun (1966). His first approximation was to consider the skin to be a semi-infinite, uniform and isotropic medium, bounded only by a plane horny layer. He further assumed that the mediating substance was formed at the junction of the horny layer and viable layer of the epidermis ($x = 0$), and instantaneously during irradiation ($t = 0$). The diffusion process is then described by the differential equation given by

$$dC(x, t)/dt = D[d^2C(x, t)/dx^2], \tag{5.1}$$

where $C(x, t)$ is the concentration of the mediator substance at a depth x normal to the skin surface and at time t after irradiation, and D is the effective diffusion coefficient. The solution of equation 5.1 which describes the spreading of the substance through the skin is

$$C(x, t) = A(Dt)^{-1/2} \exp(-x^2/4Dt), \tag{5.2}$$

where A is the total amount of mediator substance formed per unit area of skin and is assumed to be directly proportional to the UV dose. This equation was used to predict the time of appearance and disappearance of erythema as a function of UV dose. Substantial agreement between theory and observation was found with respect to 300 nm UVR erythema, though not with 250 nm UVR.

5.3.1.2 The erythema action spectrum. The ability of UVR to produce an erythema response in human skin is highly dependent upon the wavelength of the radiation and is expressed by the action spectrum. An action spectrum is a plot of the reciprocal of the dose required for a given effect against wavelength, and strictly applies only if the dose–response curves are similar at all wavelengths, which implies that the mechanism of action is the same at all wavelengths.

The erythema action spectrum has long been the subject of controversy. The first precise determination of the action spectrum was reported in 1922 and exhibited a major peak of activity at 297 nm, a minimum at 280 nm, and a second but lesser peak at 250 nm. Related studies carried out in the 1920s and 1930s showed close agreement from approximately 270 nm to 310 nm and so from these reports a 'standard erythemal curve' was adopted by the International Commission on Illumination (ICI) in 1935. This double-peaked curve was accepted as standard for many years, but more recent work in the 1960s and 1970s suggests a curve with increasing amplitude as the wavelength becomes shorter, with a 'shoulder' at about 300–280 nm. Figure 5.4 compares the ICI action spectrum with more recent estimates.

It is interesting to ask why it is that there are differences in the action spectrum determined by different workers. There are several reasons for this difference and they include the following. Firstly, it depends on when the erythema reactions are assessed; the diphasic nature of the

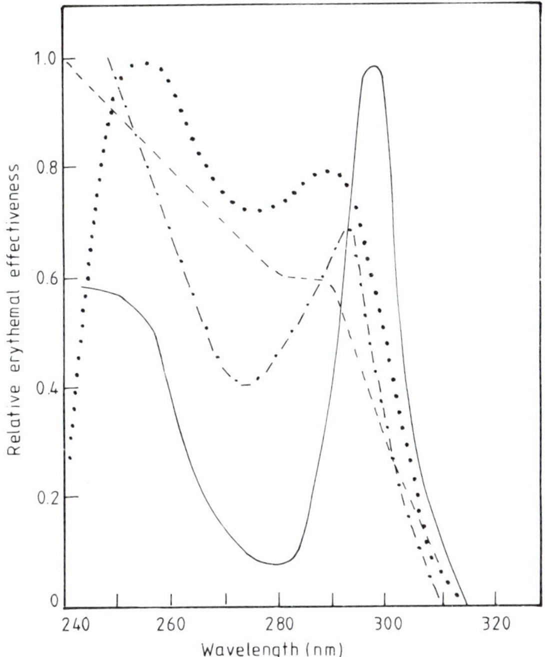

Figure 5.4 Comparison of the standard erythemal curve (ICI 1935) with the erythema action spectra determined by Everett *et al* (1965), Freeman *et al* (1966), and Cripps and Ramsay (1970): full curve, standard erythemal curve; broken curve, Everett *et al*; dotted curve, Freeman *et al*; and chain curve, Cripps and Ramsay.

curve is less obvious when observed 8 h after irradiation than at 24 h after irradiation (*see* figure 5.5). A second reason may be due to the anatomical site chosen for the irradiation; the anterior abdomen or back has been chosen in recent studies as these regions exhibit less non-uniformity in reactivity than the forearm, which was used in earlier work. Thirdly, the choice of criteria for the erythemal response is important since, as figure 5.5 illustrates, the form of the action spectrum depends upon whether the response is strictly a threshold reaction (MED) or one showing a more definite erythema.

Methods to quantify the erythemal response have involved use of both red-coloured papers and red photographic filters, with which the

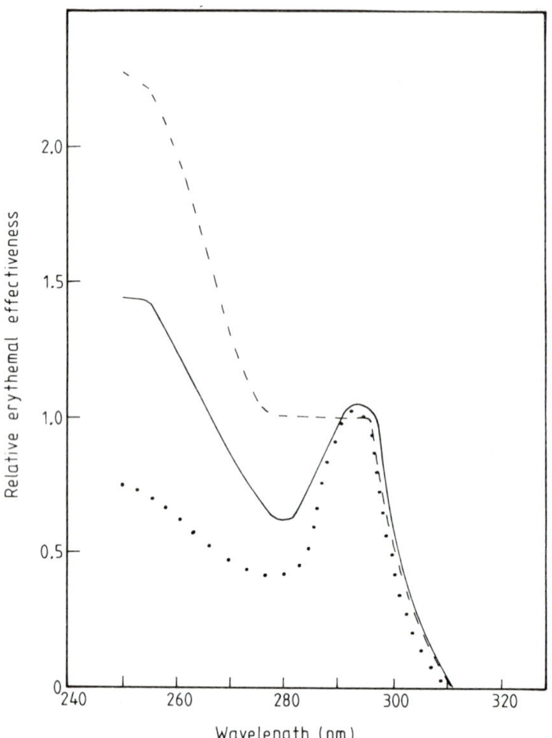

Figure 5.5 Action spectrum for human skin according to different criteria (from Berger *et al* 1968): broken curve, 8 h MED; full curve, 24 h MED; and dotted curve, 24 h moderate erythema.

reaction could be compared and graded, and also reflectance spectrophotometry. Finally, early investigations were carried out using a mercury arc lamp and quartz prism monochromator, limiting the study to those wavelengths characteristic of the mercury spectrum, whereas more recent work has utilised a xenon arc lamp and either a prism or grating monochromator, giving the investigator a choice of wavelengths from a continuous spectrum.

5.3.2 Melanin pigmentation

A socially desirable consequence of exposure to unfiltered sunlight is the delayed pigmentation of the skin known as 'tanning', which becomes noticeable about two days after exposure and gradually increases for several days. Tanning is due not only to the formation of new melanin but also to the migration of the pigment already present in the basal cells to the more superficial layers of the skin.

The familiar delayed tanning or melanogenesis may also be accompanied by immediate tanning, particularly in pigmented individuals. In general, the darker the unexposed baseline colouration, the greater is the ability to exhibit immediate tanning. Immediate tanning can become evident within 5 to 10 minutes of exposure to noonday sun and is thought to involve photo-oxidation of preformed melanin, which results in increased melanisation of melanosomes.

The threshold dose for melanogenesis and its range has not been well defined; obviously it varies considerably from one subject to another. In European stock, perhaps the threshold dose, on visual assessment, lies somewhere around 1000 $J\,m^{-2}$ for monochromatic 300 nm radiation (Magnus 1976). However, longer wavelengths than those required for erythema can produce some suntanning, even those wavelengths extending well into the UV-A and even into the visible region, although wavelengths in the UV-B region are still the most effective in initiating melanogenesis.

Once present, melanin affords protection against sunburn by decreasing the amount of UVR that can reach the lower layer of the skin, containing viable keratinocytes, or penetrate into the dermis. Studies have shown that the thickening of the epidermis that occurs after mild exposure to UVR can also afford protection against damage by UVR.

5.3.3 Production of vitamin D

The skin absorbs UV-B radiation in sunlight to convert sterol precursors in the skin, such as 7-dehydrocholesterol, to vitamin D. Vitamin D is further transformed by the liver and kidneys to biologically active metabolites such as 25-hydroxyvitamin D; these metabolites then act on the intestinal mucosa to facilitate calcium absorption, and on bone to facilitate calcium exchange.

It has long been recognised that children chronically under-exposed to adequate amounts of solar UVR may develop rickets, a deforming disease characterised by under-mineralisation of the bones. The disease can be cured by exposure to natural or artificial sources of UVR incorporating wavelengths less than 315 nm. The antirachitic efficiency of UVR as a function of wavelength is shown in figure 5.6.

The long-wavelength limit for the antirachitic action spectrum is

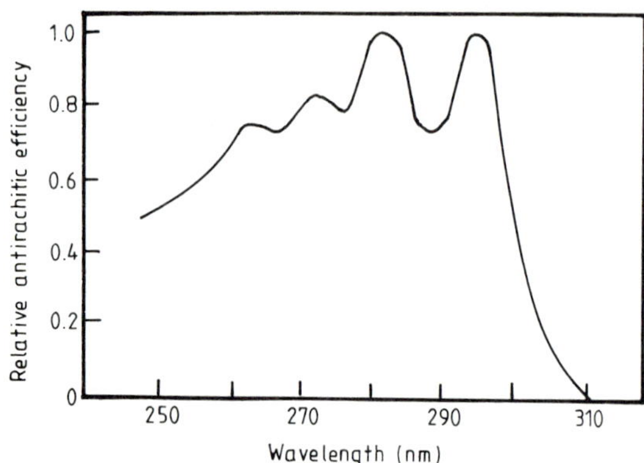

Figure 5.6 Antirachitic action spectrum (after Bachem 1956).

approximately the same as the erythema action spectrum (*see* figure 5.4), whereas the maximum of the antirachitic curve occurs at 280 nm, which corresponds to the minimum, or shoulder, of the erythema curve.

Suberythemal doses of UV-B are sufficient for the satisfactory synthesis of vitamin D; the amount of sunlight received during a 15 minute lunchtime walk during the summer is enough. However because of the low levels of UV-B received by the population in winter months, it is not uncommon for normal healthy persons living in northern latitudes to develop an impairment in the ability of their intestinal mucosa to absorb calcium during this period. This impairment could be prevented if they were exposed to an artificial light source which emitted small quantities of UV-B.

5.3.4 Ageing of the skin

Chronic exposure to sunlight can result in an appearance of the skin often referred to as premature ageing or actinic damage. The clinical changes associated with skin ageing include a dry, coarse, leathery appearance, laxity with wrinkling, and various pigmentary changes. Light-skinned Caucasians are more susceptible to sun damage than Negroes, since the black skin of the latter affords more natural protection because of its high melanin content. Skin ageing is probably best characterised by the peasant population of Mediterranean races who spend many years outdoors in hot sunshine. It is particularly a problem in

Israel where, following the last World War, large numbers of North European and Russian Jews settled. Unlike the Arabs in surrounding countries, however, their skin has not yet adapted to the intense solar radiation environment of the Middle East. Perhaps with the recent increase in the availability of whole body UV irradiation for cosmetic purposes we may well see similar skin appearances in people in our own country.

5.3.5 The carcinogenic nature of ultraviolet radiation

The idea that chronic exposure to sunlight is a cause of skin cancer is not an old one. The earliest suggestions appear to have come in 1894 from the dermatologist Unna who referred to a precancerous development which he coined as 'Seaman's Skin'. Since then it has gradually been accepted that sunlight, or more precisely those wavelengths less than about 320 nm, plays an aetiological role in the formation of skin cancer in man. There appears to be little question now that the majority of squamous cell carcinomas are caused by chronic exposure to sunlight, although such a clear relationship between the incidence of either basal cell carcinomas or, more particularly, malignant melanoma and sunlight exposure has not been demonstrated.

The evidence for the carcinogenic effects of UVR is of different kinds, some of it more convincing than others, but all converging.

(1) There is strong evidence in the anatomical distribution of skin cancers, which in light-complexioned peoples appear predominantly on areas not ordinarily protected by hair or clothing. It has been demonstrated that about 90% of all basal cell carcinomas and more than half of all squamous cell carcinomas occur on the head and neck. Studies made comparing the geometry of insolation of the head and neck areas with sites of non-melanoma cancers indicate that two thirds of basal cell carcinomas and virtually all squamous cell carcinomas occur on the skin sites receiving the highest doses of UVR. The anatomical distribution of malignant melanoma, a less common but more lethal form of skin cancer, suggests a less striking association with exposure to UVR. However, there has been an increased prevalence of this type of cancer on the legs of women during the past 25 years, suggesting an association with the fashion for shorter skirts.

(2) Negroes are notably free from skin cancer, this corresponding to their relative insensitivity to sunburn. Both factors may be accounted for, in part at least, by the greater opacity of the horny layer of the

epidermis. This greater opacity may be due to greater thickness of the horny layer, as well as to a greater amount of melanin, although the exact role of this pigment is not clear, and correlation of sunburn or skin cancer with skin colour is not to be trusted.

(3) It is widely accepted that persons who are much exposed to solar UVR because of occupation are more likely to get skin cancer. Although this generalisation seems sound enough, it must be admitted that statistics to establish it beyond question are lacking. Nevertheless data exist which demonstrate that farmers, fishermen, sailors, and others such as road workers, policemen and postmen have a higher incidence of skin cancer than office and factory workers.

(4) In general, the incidence of skin cancer is highest in fair-skinned people who live in tropical and sub-tropical areas. This corresponds to the high levels of solar UV-B encountered in these areas, since it is this part of the global spectrum which is believed to be responsible for skin carcinogenesis. However, incidence data for skin cancer, other than melanoma, must be treated with caution, since many cancer registries do not keep records of non-melanoma skin cancer.

(5) People suffering from the skin disease, *xeroderma pigmentosum* (XP), due to an hereditary defect, show abnormal pigmentation and high incidence of skin cancers initiated by exposure to solar UVR. There is evidence of some correlation between the clinical severity of the symptoms in these patients and the degree of impairment of DNA repair provoked by UVR exposure. Reduction of DNA repair in XP patients could very plausibly be related to carcinogenesis.

(6) Perhaps the most convincing evidence comes from laboratory experiments; skin cancer can be induced in mice and rats with repeated doses of UVR. The upper wavelength limit of the effective cancer-producing radiation is about 320 nm, which is the same spectral range producing erythema in human skin.

5.3.5.1 The carcinogenic action spectrum. It is, of course, not possible to determine experimentally the action spectrum for skin carcinogenesis in man. Nevertheless it is widely believed that only those wavelengths less than 320 nm are responsible. This belief arises from three sources: results of experiments in animal photocarcinogenesis; observations on the geographical distribution of non-melanoma skin cancers in man; and the hypothesis that the molecule deoxyribonucleic acid (DNA) is the target for UV-induced carcinogenesis.

Precise determination of the action spectrum for non-melanoma tumour induction in animals, notably hairless mice, has not been accomplished because of the problems associated with methodology. The factors involved in such a study include the large number of potential wavelengths; the need for monochromators with extremely low levels of stray radiation; the considerable number of experimental animals required, together with problems of immobilisation; and, not least, the length of time (a matter of months or even years) required for exposure to each wavelength. Notwithstanding these difficulties, the action spectrum for photocarcinogenesis in mice appears to be similar to that for induction of delayed erythema; that is, restricted to wavelengths less than 320 nm. Recent work has demonstrated that UV-A, in doses of the same order of magnitude as that existing in sunlight, is not carcinogenic for mouse skin. Also the presence of UV-A in a spectrum also containing UV-B does not appear to enhance the carcinogenic effect of UV-B alone.

It has previously been mentioned that skin cancers in man tend to increase with environmental levels of UV-B. This relationship will be covered in more detail in the next section on dose–response models.

Finally, it cannot be assumed that the action spectra for erythema and cancer in human skin are similar unless a common chromophore or action mechanism is involved. In 1974 Setlow proposed that the common denominator was the action spectrum for affecting DNA since there is overwhelming evidence that changes in DNA—for example, formation of pyrimidine dimers and other photochemical products—have important biological consequences, such as the killing of cells and the induction of mutations. By taking into account the transmission of UVR in skin, he showed that the shapes of action spectra for DNA, erythema, and possibly skin cancer production were similar, and could be made to coincide.

5.3.5.2 Models of skin photocarcinogenesis. At present there are no firm data on the relationship between incidence of skin tumours and UVR exposure. Neither the appropriate dose rate nor what the induction time might be is known in the case of human skin cancer apparently provoked by sunlight.

There is ample evidence that a geographical latitude gradient exists for the incidence of skin cancer in sun-sensitive, fair-skinned populations, and that this gradient is non-linear. Correlation of observed ultraviolet exposure and skin cancer incidence in Australia resulted in the finding that in going from Brisbane (latitude 27 °S) to Cloncurry (21 °S) an increase of roughly three times the skin tumour frequency corresponded to an exposure increase of wavelengths less than 320 nm of about 1.5–1.6, which suggests that tumour incidence is proportional to the square of the environmental UV dose. Furthermore, from detailed epidemiological investigations, Urbach and his colleagues (1974) have estimated that the incidence of skin cancer approximately doubles for every 10 degrees decrease of latitude, provided that the population is of reasonably similar genetic stock. Calculations have shown that the erythemally effective, and presumably carcinogenic, global UV radiation increases with the square of decrease in latitude, and so this result, coupled with Urbach's estimate, leads to a rather complex relationship between skin cancer incidence and sunlight exposure.

More recently the ultraviolet dose dependence of non-melanoma skin cancer incidence has been studied by Green *et al* (1976) and Fears *et al* (1977). These authors have correlated epidemiological skin cancer data with both measured and calculated estimates of the UV environment. In both instances the age-adjusted data have been modelled by a power law relationship of the form

$$\text{skin cancer incidence} \propto (\text{annual UV dose})^p. \quad (5.3)$$

A power law representation of age-adjusted incidence data versus UV dose has the convenience that the power p serves as a constant 'biological amplification factor' in the sense that

$$p = (\mathrm{d}I/I)/(\mathrm{d}D/D), \quad (5.4)$$

where I is skin cancer incidence and D is annual UV dose. Green *et al* (1976) have found that p varies from 0.0 ± 2.0 to 3.8 ± 2.0, depending upon geographical location, although a consolidated fit to the complete ensemble of data led to a value of $p = 2.5 \pm 0.3$. Fears *et al* (1977) obtained values of p equal to 2.96 ± 0.59 and 2.45 ± 0.63 for non-melanoma skin cancer in males and females respectively. These authors correlated the incidence of skin cancer among white people in the United States using data contained in the Third National Cancer Survey (Cutler and Young 1975), with field measurements of biologically effective UVR at ten locations in the USA.

However, in 1978 Green pointed out that the spectral response of the Robertson–Berger UV meter used in this survey falls off more slowly at longer wavelengths than the DNA action spectrum which is thought to be the relevant biophysical mechanism for skin cancer. By appropriate correction of the UV dose measurements of Fears *et al* (1977), Green has concluded that the risk of non-melanoma skin cancer depends upon a factor of UV dose raised to the power of 1.8.

While it is evident that the uncertainties associated with the conclusions of these studies are large, the best accepted model data to date suggest that a 5% increase in erythemally effective global UVR may result in a 15% (range 7.5–25%) increase in skin cancer in a susceptible population after about 60 years, when a steady state has been reached.

5.4 Photodermatoses

A photodermatosis is a skin disease which is either light-induced or aggravated by light. A distinction may be made between primary and secondary photosensitive conditions. Primary photosensitivity includes such diseases as polymorphic light eruption, actinic reticuloid and solar urticaria. In secondary photosensitivity the condition may be the result of some other disease such as porphyria, or of recognisable external factors such as drugs or chemicals which may be therapeutic, cosmetic, industrial, and so on.

5.4.1 Primary photosensitivity

5.4.1.1 Polymorphic light eruption. This is a common photodermatosis of unknown aetiology. The age of onset can be very variable although it usually appears in the second and third decades. Once present the disease seems to be recurrent and can last an indefinite number of years. As the name suggests there may be a variety of morphological lesions on light-exposed areas, for example, erythema, eczema, papules, plaques or blisters. The latent period between exposure and appearance of the rash lies between a few hours to two days. Attacks generally start in the spring and continue through until winter. There is, however, a tendency in some patients for the eruptions to subside in the summer. The site of eruption depends upon sunlight exposure of unclothed areas although the most favoured sites are the backs of the hands, the front of the neck and the face.

The action spectrum for the disease lies in the normal sunburn range for most patients, although some patients may react with UV-A radiation. Also many patients exhibit abnormal morphological responses with doses in excess of the MED in the 300 nm region.

5.4.1.2 Actinic reticuloid. This is a condition of unknown aetiology occurring in middle aged or elderly men who commonly have a long history of chronic skin disease, e.g. psoriasis, contact dermatitis. The rash is not necessarily confined to sun-exposed sites and lesions can extend onto covered areas. Morphologically the lesions may resemble that of a chronic erythematous, erythemato-vascular, or erythemato-squamous dermatitis accompanied by thickening of the skin and lichenification.

Photobiological tests show a markedly increased abnormal reactivity over a wide spectrum extending from below 300 nm up to at least 360 nm and not uncommonly to about 600 nm. The MED can be as low as 10 $J\,m^{-2}$ at 300 nm and 5000 $J\,m^{-2}$ in the UV-A. Test exposures in both the UV-B and UV-A often produce erythematous swellings, although responses to visible radiation tend to be erythematous without swelling. There is a latent period of between 6 and 18 hours after exposure before a response is evident.

5.4.1.3 Solar urticaria. Unlike the previous two photodermatoses, solar urticaria evolves during or within a few minutes of irradiation and usually resolves within half an hour. Erythema localised to the exposed skin site appears first and may be accompanied by a sensation of itching or burning. This is followed by the development of a weal which reaches its greatest extent in about 5–10 min.

Because of the very rapid evolution of the lesion in solar urticaria, it is relatively easy to investigate with a monochromator, although classification of an action spectrum has proved difficult. In fact there does not appear to be a definitive action spectrum; different groups have reacted in the UV-B, UV-A, visible spectrum around 500 nm, and even in a more or less continuum from 250–700 nm.

5.4.2 Secondary photosensitivity

5.4.2.1 Porphyria. Porphyria is the collective name given to a rare group of hereditary disorders associated with abnormalities in haem biosynthesis. A manifestation of the disease is the excessive production of porphyrins, which appear in the urine either as red pigments or as colourless compounds that darken on exposure to light. One of the clinical symptoms of porphyria is skin photosensitivity, which may be evident at an early age.

In acid solution porphyrins of clinical interest have strong absorption spectra, especially in the region near 400 nm (the so-called Soret band). In a neutral pH system such as the skin the Soret peak is broadened, but nevertheless the skin of a porphyric patient irradiated with a

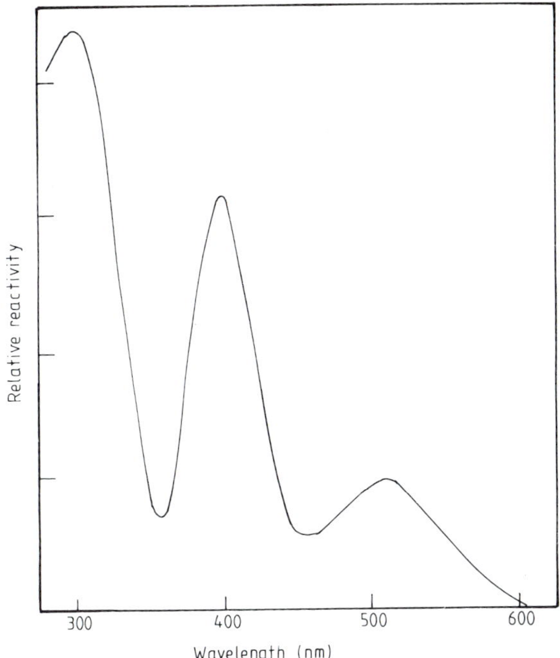

Figure 5.7 Action spectrum for skin photosensitivity which is typical in a highly photosensitive patient with porphyria.

monochromator may show increased reactivity at wavelengths around 400 nm (*see* figure 5.7).

Porphyric photosensitivity may manifest itself as subjective symptoms, often of a 'burning' character, during or soon after exposure to sunlight, and skin changes such as erythema or oedema which can appear within an hour or up to 18 hours after exposure.

5.4.2.2 Drug and chemical photosensitivity. Chemicals which cause photosensitisation may enter the body by ingestion, injection or absorption through the skin. The speed of effect and severity of the symptoms depend upon the route of entry. In general, topical substances like pitch, tar or synthetic dyes give symptoms such as erythema or oedema which can occur within minutes of exposure to the sun. Orally administered photosensitisers, such as therapeutic drugs, will not produce symptoms until an effective concentration is present in the skin and this may take several days or weeks. The principal reaction is erythema, although symptoms such as a bullous eruption may occur with some drugs, e.g. nalidixic acid. Some common chemical photosensitisers are listed in table 5.2.

Table 5.2 Some common chemical photosensitisers.

Hypnotics	e.g. phenobarbitone
Tranquillisers	e.g. phenothiazines, especially chlorpromazine
Diuretics	e.g. thiazides
Antibiotics	e.g. tetracyclines
Sulphonamides	e.g. sulphamethoxazole with trimethoprim
Antibacterials	e.g. nalidixic acid
Oral contraceptives†	
Sunscreens	
Tar	
Cosmetics, due to presence of eosin or psoralens, for example.	

† It is uncertain whether these drugs result in photosensitivity in some people.

The action spectrum in the skin of a photosensitiser may be similar to its absorption spectrum *in vitro*. Demethylchloretetracycline and sometimes chlorpromazine may act in this way. However the photosensitiser may often metabolise in the body so that the absorption and action spectra may differ. A well-known example of this latter process is in the psoralens where the action spectrum is the consequence of psoralens forming a photoadduct with DNA. The absorption spectrum of psoralens decreases in amplitude as the wavelength increases above 300 nm, yet psoralen photosensitisation occurs in the UV-A.

5.5 Structure of the Eye

A schematic sagittal section of the human eye is illustrated in figure 5.8. The eye is almost spherical, approximately one inch in diameter, but with a more acutely convex bulge at the front formed by the cornea. The neurophysiological responses to photons in the visible region of the electromagnetic spectrum are relayed to the brain via the optic nerve at the back of the eye. The eyeball consists of three co-spherical layers.

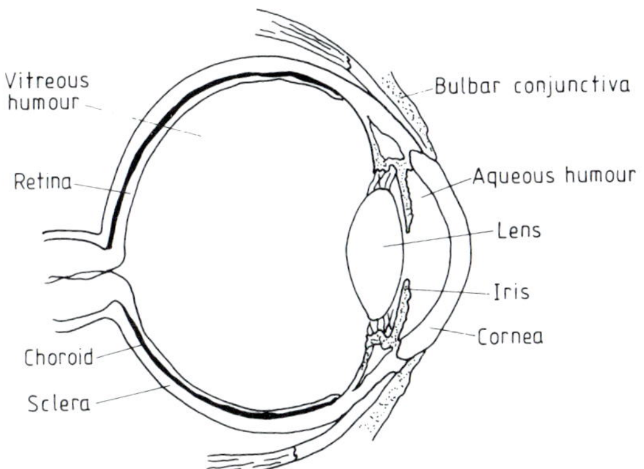

Figure 5.8 Schematic structure of the human eye.

(1) An outer protective sclera, the opaque white of the eye surrounding the whole globe apart from where it merges into the cornea. The air–cornea interface represents the principal refracting boundary in the eye.

(2) An intermediate pigmented layer termed the choroid which is modified in front to form the iris diaphragm of variable aperture immediately in front of the lens.

(3) An internal nervous layer, the retina, adapted for the reception of light stimuli.

Within the eye there are three different types of refracting medium:

(a) the watery aqueous humour which fills the space between the lens and the cornea;

(b) the translucent solid lens, which can be modified in curvature so as to accommodate for near and far vision; and

(c) the thin jelly of the vitreous humour which fills the bulk of the eye.

5.6 Ultraviolet Optics of the Eye

Most of the measurements on the ultraviolet transmission through the eye have been performed in animals, notably in the rabbit eye. This section, however, discusses UV transmission through the human eye from measurements carried out by Boettner and Wolter (1962).

These investigators studied the optical properties of nine normal human eyes taken from patients varying in age from 4 weeks to 75 years during surgical operation. Immediately after enucleation of the eye it was divided into its components. The aqueous humour and vitreous humour were withdrawn with a hypodermic needle and syringe and transferred to quartz cuvettes. The cornea and lens were removed by dissection. Each component was placed in turn at the entrance aperture of an integrating sphere housed in a spectrophotometer so as to measure total transmittance, i.e. direct plus scattered radiation. Figure 5.9 illustrates the average fraction of UVR incident on the aqueous humour, the lens, and the vitreous humour. These data have been estimated from the spectral transmittance curves for each component given by Boettner and Wolter. Two points are worth noting. Ultraviolet radiation with wavelength less than 310 nm is absorbed mainly in the cornea. This corresponds to the observation that acute biological effects of UV exposure to the eye are limited to the UV-B and UV-C and occur predominantly

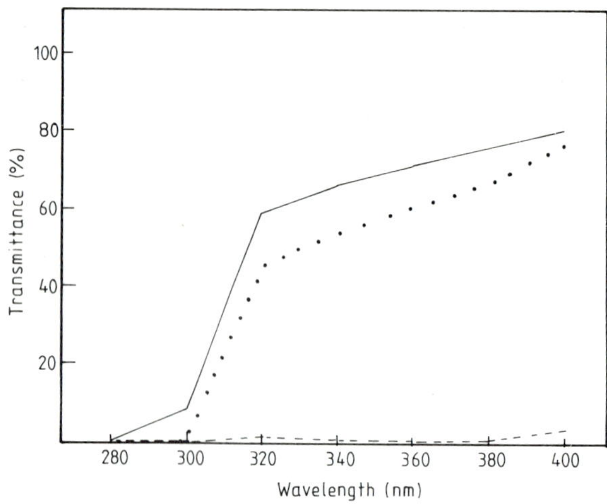

Figure 5.9 Average fraction of UVR incident on the aqueous humour (full curve), the lens (dotted curve) and the vitreous humour (broken curve) of the human eye (after Boettner and Wolter 1962).

in the corneal tissue. Secondly, UV-A radiation is absorbed primarily in the lens, which supports the hypothesis that UV-A may be implicated in the production of cataracts.

5.7 Effects of Ultraviolet Radiation on the Eye

5.7.1 Photokeratitis and conjunctivitis

The acute effects of exposure to UV-C and UV-B radiation are primarily those of conjunctivitis and photokeratitis.

Conjunctivitis is an inflammation of the membrane that lines the insides of the eyelids and covers the cornea, and may often be accompanied by an erythema of the skin around the eyelids. There is the sensation of 'sand in the eyes' and also varying degrees of photophobia (aversion to light), lacrimation (tears), and blepharospasm (spasm of the eyelid muscles) may be present.

Photokeratitis is an inflammation of the cornea which can result in severe pain. Ordinary clinical photokeratitis is characterised by a period of latency that tends to vary inversely with the severity of UV exposure. The latent period may be as short as 30 min or as long as 24 h, but it is typically 6–12 h. The acute symptoms of visual incapacitation usually last from 6–24 h. Almost all discomfort disappears within two days and rarely does exposure result in permanent damage. Unlike the skin, the ocular system does not develop tolerance to repeated exposure to UVR. Many cases of photokeratitis have been reported following exposure to UVR produced by welding arcs and by the reflection of solar radiation from snow and sand. For this reason the condition is sometimes referred to as 'welders flash', 'arc eye', or 'snow blindness'.

5.7.1.1 Action spectrum for corneal effects. There have been several attempts to define an ultraviolet ocular action spectrum, but in general corneal damage has been taken as the end point for most studies of wavelengths less than 320 nm. Most published data on ocular action spectra have been obtained by using the rabbit as the experimental model, although results have also been reported for primates and for man. Criteria used to establish a threshold response have included the appearance of some or all of the following:

(a) epithelial debris—small glistening bodies located in the pre-corneal tear layer;

(b) epithelial haze—an irregular, crackled appearance of the anterior surface of the cornea;

(c) epithelial granules—small, white, discrete, round spots located deep in the epithelial layer of the cornea; and

(d) photophobia—avoidance response to light.

A comparison of the radiant exposure thresholds for rabbits, primates and man is shown in figure 5.10. The data were obtained by Pitts and his colleagues using a xenon lamp and grating monochromator and were established by irradiating 238 rabbit eyes, 83 primate eyes and 39 human eyes. Note that for all three species the minimum threshold occurs at a wavelength of 270 nm and a radiant exposure of 40 $J\,m^{-2}$.

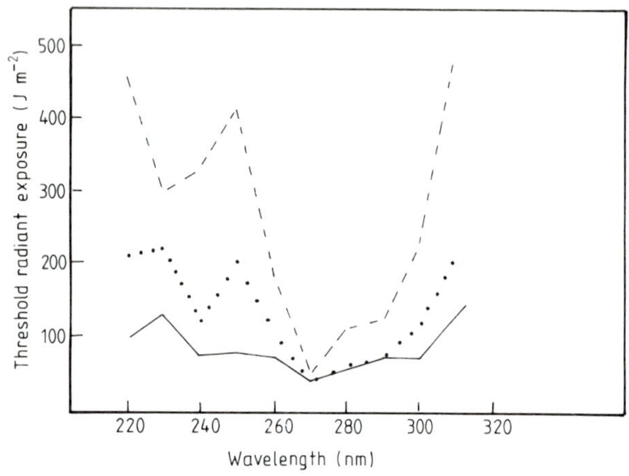

Figure 5.10 Comparison of the radiant exposure thresholds for the cornea of the human (full curve), the primate (dotted curve), and the rabbit (broken curve) (from Pitts 1973).

5.7.2 Cataracts

A cataract is a partial or complete loss of transparency of the lens or its capsule. Most of the available data on the production of cataracts have been obtained using the rabbit. The most effective wavelengths for producing lenticular opacities appear to lie in the range 295–315 nm.

Chemical effects in the lens protein, tryptophan, have been shown to occur after UV-A exposure of human crystalline lenses. The effects lead to the formation of chromatic photoproducts that bind to, and alter, the solubility of lens proteins, resulting in a yellowing of the lens material. While the basic biochemical mechanisms remain to be found, it is nevertheless suggested that exposure to UV-A can enhance cataractogenesis in humans.

There is scant evidence that the incidence of cataracts is increased in temperate areas and is more common in outdoor, rather than indoor workers. Although circumstantial evidence does not prove a relationship between sunlight exposure and human cataracts, the evidence does suggest a causal relationship to be a likely possibility.

One of the current applications of UVR in medicine is so-called psoralen photochemotherapy, or PUVA, for the treatment of certain skin diseases (*see* § 6.3). In this treatment patients are orally administered the phototoxic derivative, 8-methoxypsoralen, and shortly afterwards exposed to UV-A. It is known that such compounds can cuase UV-A induced corneal opacities and cataracts in experimental animals, although the mechanism of ocular photosensitisation by psoralens is uncertain. Clearly the need for verification and understanding of the ocular effects that may be produced in humans by the combination of UV-A and photosensitising drugs is apparent.

6 Medical Applications of Ultraviolet Radiation

Ultraviolet radiation has a variety of applications in medicine under headings which can be broadly classified as therapy, diagnosis and non-clinical applications. It is difficult to summarise the current status of ultraviolet radiation in medicine; its use in physiotherapy has certainly diminished in recent years, but the combination of ultraviolet radiation with photoactive drugs is now the treatment of choice for many skin diseases. The diagnosis of abnormal photosensitivity is increasingly achieved by combining the results of detailed photobiological investigations with clinical examination. These and other current applications of UVR in medicine will be discussed in this chapter.

6.1 The Use of Ultraviolet Radiation in Physiotherapy

The therapeutic use of UVR, or actinotherapy as it is sometimes called, is no more evident in medicine than in the physiotherapy department. In its time, actinotherapy has been used to treat a host of various disorders, including anthrax, carbon monoxide poisoning, diabetes, heart and lung diseases, as well as numerous skin diseases. In particular, actinotherapy and heliotherapy have proved extremely beneficial in the treatment of tuberculosis, although the advent of antibiotics and the greater awareness of the importance of public health have now made the treatment obsolete. As medical science has progressed many of these treatments have fallen into disuse, either because they were based upon unsound scientific principles or else have succumbed to more effective therapy using drugs and so on. Nevertheless UVR still remains a valuable therapeutic agent for a limited number of disorders and this section will concern itself with those conditions which are currently treated by the physiotherapist.

6.1.1 UV dosimetry in physiotherapy

It is the custom in actinotherapy to use the patient as his own biological monitor. Before embarking upon a course of irradiation small areas of the patient's skin are exposed for varying times to the radiation from the lamp to be used for treatment, at the appropriate distance. The time that is sufficient to produce a just perceptible reddening is noted and so the exposure necessary for any other degree of erythema can be determined as discussed below.

The erythema reaction following exposure to UVR is classified into one of four categories, depending upon the severity of the reaction.

(1) *First degree erythema* (E_1)—a just perceptible erythema, often referred to as the minimal erythema dose (MED), which lasts for about 24 h and leaves the skin apparently unchanged.

(2) *Second degree erythema* (E_2)—a response resembling a mild sunburn which subsides after 3–4 d and may be followed by tanning.

(3) *Third degree erythema* (E_3)—a severe reaction in which the erythema is accompanied by oedema and tenderness. The reaction lasts for several days, pigmentation is more apparent and exfoliation is marked; the skin often peels off in sheets or flakes.

(4) *Fourth degree erythema* (E_4)—the initial changes are the same as in an E_3 reaction, but the oedema and exudation are so severe that a blister is formed.

As a rough guide, the relative exposure times needed to produce an E_1 through to an E_4 are in the ratio 1:2.5:5:10. Since it is not the general practice to employ instrumentation in dosimetry, the physiotherapist will often make simple calculations based upon the inverse square law—for example, to determine a treatment time if the skin testing has been performed at a distance other than the treatment distance.

6.1.2 Clinical uses of actinotherapy

Ultraviolet radiation may be prescribed to obtain one or more of the following effects: stimulation of the skin; vitamin D production; counter-irritation; sterilisation; production of pigmentation; and exfoliation of the skin. The radiation may be administered as contact therapy (with the Kromayer lamp), regional therapy (with the Alpine sunlamp), or generalised therapy (with banks of fluorescent UV-B sunlamps). The main indications for actinotherapy nowadays are in the treatment of certain skin diseases and of superficial ulcers. The two skin diseases which respond most readily to UVR therapy are psoriasis and acne, whilst other conditions which are sometimes treated by this technique are chilblains and, more rarely, impetigo, alopecia and eczema.

6.1.2.1 Psoriasis. The preferred method of treatment for psoriasis is to use the UVR in conjunction with a photosensitiser, and these techniques are discussed in § 6.2 and § 6.3. It is rare these days for the disease to be controlled by ultraviolet irradiation alone in a physiotherapy department.

6.1.2.2 Acne. Acne vulgaris is an excessive activity of the sebaceous (grease) glands resulting in blockage by sebum (*see* figure 6.1). The condition often responds well to ultraviolet irradiation, the object being to cause exfoliation of the superficial layers of the skin which allows the sebum easier exit. The technique is to produce a first to second degree erythema so as to result in exfoliation with minimal discomfort to the patient. Particular care must be exercised when treating the face, for cosmetic reasons.

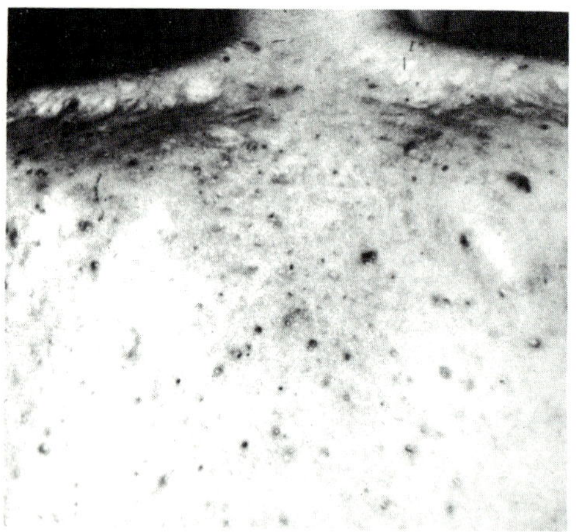

Figure 6.1 A patient with acne vulgaris.

6.1.2.3 Chilblains. Chilblains result from an exaggerated response to cold in which the blood vessels of the skin contract so much that the skin is deprived of blood and oxygen. This causes swelling, itching and a characteristic burning sensation, usually confined to the fingers and toes. The principal aim of actinotherapy is to achieve repeated first degree erythema on the affected parts in order to stimulate blood supply, although this is one example of a disease where prevention, by keeping the sensitive areas warm, is much more effective than treatment.

6.1.2.4 Ulcers. Ultraviolet irradiation of ulcers is often of considerable value and has been practiced in physiotherapy for several years. The success of the treatment relies upon the bactericidal properties of UVR and for this reason it is important that the lamp emit UV-C radiation (*see* figure 6.8). The lamp of choice is invariably the Kromayer lamp since it combines UV-C emission with a short treatment distance, resulting in a high irradiance and consequently a reasonable exposure time for the very high doses required in treating the ulcer. The procedure is to irradiate the floor of the ulcer with 20–100 times the dose required for a first degree erythema. An area of 1–2 mm of the epithelial edge of the ulcer is included in the irradiation field so as to stimulate the process of repair. Indolent ulcers will start to heal in about 5–7 days following irradiation.

6.2 Phototherapy of Psoriasis

Psoriasis is a common skin disease which affects between 1 and 2% of the population. The most usual form of psoriasis is known as plaque psoriasis and is characterised by well demarcated red plaques with a silvery scale (*see* figure 6.2). Other less common forms of the disease include flexural, scalp, guttate, erythrodermic and pustular psoriasis. The aetiology of the disease is still uncertain, although a genetic factor is involved in about one-third of patients. Other factors which influence the exacerbation of psoriasis include trauma; streptococcal infection; emotional stress; climatic factors, particularly sunlight; hormonal disturbance; and drug eruption. The clinical manifestations of psoriasis are mostly accounted for by the increased rate of mitosis in the epidermis, in which the turnover rate is 2–5 d as compared with about 25–28 d in normal skin.

The standard treatment for psoriasis is usually ultraviolet irradiation in conjunction with a topical photosensitiser. The two most common photosensitisers which have been widely used for many years are tar and dithranol.

In the so-called Goeckerman regimen, a total-body application of crude coal tar in petrolatum is applied 2–3 times a day. Each morning the tar is removed and the patient is irradiated in either a cubicle containing banks of UV-B fluorescent sunlamps or by a medium-pressure

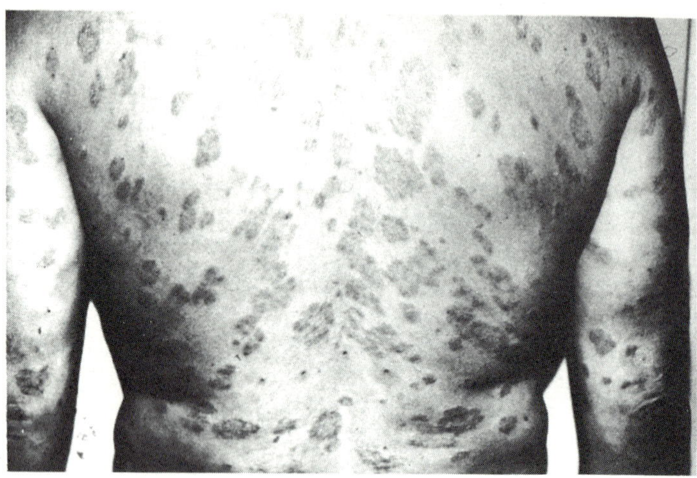

Figure 6.2 A patient with plaque psoriasis.

mercury vapour lamp, such as the Alpine sunlamp. The exposure time is such as to maintain a second degree erythema. After ultraviolet treatment the patient bathes, the tar is reapplied 2–3 times during the day and the patient is irradiated again the following morning. The exposure times must be increased as the patient tans and his stratum corneum thickens, resulting in daily UV-B treatment doses in the range 100–5000 $J\,m^{-2}$. The Goeckerman regimen demands hospitalisation of the patient for two to three weeks, although severe cases may require up to seven weeks in hospital. The average length of remission following treatment is around two years.

Although the Goeckerman regimen has been practised for 55 years and is one of the most effective forms of therapy available for psoriasis, the mechanism of the treatment still remains obscure. The action spectrum for the regression of psoriatic lesions is unknown but it is established that both UV-A and UV-B are equally therapeutic when using exposures adequate to cause cutaneous phototoxicity. Since the daily dose of UV-A must be in the range 3×10^5–$3 \times 10^6\ J\,m^{-2}$ to benefit tar-treated skin, currently available light sources are impractical to deliver these high doses, and so UV-B sources are still the lamps of choice.

The disadvantages of tar include its mess, its smell, its irritancy and its carcinogenicity, and for these reasons British dermatological practice generally favours a modification of the Goeckerman regimen, known as the Ingram regimen, for the treatment of plaque psoriasis. In this regimen the patient has a tar bath followed by exposure to UV-B from either fluorescent sunlamps or a medium-pressure mercury vapour lamp. Dithranol (a synthetic substance that inhibits DNA synthesis), at a concentration of 0.05–0.5% in Lassar's paste, is carefully applied to the psoriatic lesions only and covered with bandages or tube gauze. This treatment is repeated daily for two or three weeks, when the psoriasis will be cleared in the majority of patients. The length of time before relapse is comparable with that obtained in the Goeckerman regimen.

An intriguing form of phototherapy for psoriasis is that experienced by patients who bask in the sun by the side of the Dead Sea in Israel. Considerable relief has been experienced by many patients, so much so that many Danish dermatologists prefer to send patients there for four week periods rather than admit them to hospital. Certainly there are economic as well as medical benefits in prescribing this form of therapy.

Again, the mechanism of treatment is poorly understood. The Dead Sea is 400 m below sea level and measurements of the solar spectral irradiance on the shores of the Dead Sea have yielded a much lower UV-B component than recorded at other sites in Israel. This means that patients are able to tolerate much longer exposures to the sun without the risk of sunburn. Also, the Dead Sea has a rich abundance of minerals and organic substances amongst which may be an efficient photosensitising material. Finally, it should be commented that the beauty of the surroundings, the clear blue skies and the total tranquillity may all play some role in helping the patient relax and perhaps aid in the regression of the disease.

6.3 Psoralen Photochemotherapy

Probably the most exciting development of the use of ultraviolet radiation in clinical medicine in recent years has been psoralen photochemotherapy. This form of treatment, known colloquially as PUVA, involves the combination of the photoactive drugs, psoralens (P), with long wave ultraviolet radiation (UV-A) to produce a beneficial effect. Psoralen photochemotherapy has been used to treat many skin diseases in the past decade, although its principal success has been in the management of psoriasis, a disorder characterised by an accelerated cell cycle and rate of DNA synthesis. The mechanism of the treatment is thought to be that psoralens bind to DNA in the presence of UV-A, resulting in a subsequent transient inhibition of DNA synthesis and cell division. The psoralens may be applied to the skin either topically or systemically; the latter route is generally preferred and the psoralens are administered as 8-methoxypsoralen (8-MOP).

6.3.1 Treatment regimen

The patient ingests the 8-MOP tablets and, two hours later, when the photosensitivity of the skin is at a maximum, he is exposed to UV-A radiation. If the psoriasis is generalised, whole body exposure is given in the type of irradiation cabinet shown in figure 6.3. This unit incorporates 48 high-intensity UV-A fluorescent lamps with the spectral power distribution shown in figure 2.9. Although this type of lamp is by far the most common source of UV-A in photochemotherapy, other lamps which have been successfully used include dysprosium lamps (Fischer and Alsins 1976), metal halide lamps (Fry 1977), and a filtered, medium-

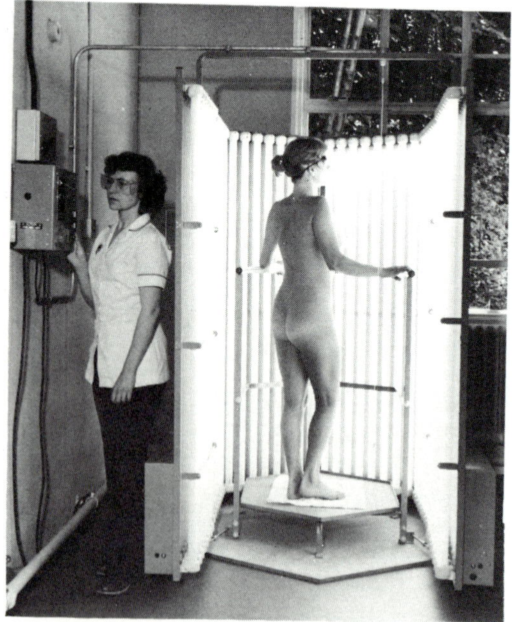

Figure 6.3 A whole body UV-A irradiation cubicle. (Courtesy of Rank Stanley Cox, Ware, UK.)

pressure, mercury-vapour lamp in which the patient rotates in front of a single high-intensity linear lamp (Diffey and Keir 1977). The initial UV-A radiant exposure (in $J\,m^{-2}$) will depend upon the spectral power distribution of the source and the skin type of the patient. This starting dose is determined either from the criteria in table 6.1 or by evaluating the minimal photoxicity dose; small areas of psoralen sensitised skin are irradiated with increasing exposures of UV-A and that dose which produces a barely perceptible, well-defined erythema 72 h later is taken as the initial dose. The radiant exposure is increased at regular intervals throughout the course of treatment to keep pace with increasing melanisation. The exposure time may vary from a few minutes to up to an hour, depending upon the above factors and also on the irradiance at the patient's skin, which reflects the design of the treatment cubicle. Values of UV-A irradiance in clinical treatment cubicles have been found to range from 16–140 $W\,m^{-2}$, although an irradiance of 50 $W\,m^{-2}$ is probably typical.

Table 6.1 Initial UV-A radiant exposures for patients embarking on PUVA therapy.

Skin Type	Criteria	$J\,m^{-2}$
I	Always burn, never tan	1.5×10^4
II	Always burn, sometimes tan	2.5×10^4
III	Somtimes burn, always tan	3.5×10^4
IV	Never burn, always tan	4.5×10^4
V	Moderately pigmented subjects e.g. Arabs	5.5×10^4
VI	Heavily pigmented subjects e.g. Negroes	6.5×10^4

Treatment is given two or three times weekly until the psoriasis clears. The total time taken for this to occur will obviously vary considerably from one patient to another, and in some cases complete clearing of the lesions is never achieved. However it would be fair to say that something like 25 treatments are required for clearing of the psoriatic lesions in most patients over a period of around 10 weeks. PUVA therapy is not a cure for psoriasis and maintenance therapy is often needed at intervals of, say, once a week to once a month to prevent relapse. Since the encouraging results of PUVA therapy for psoriasis were first reported by Parrish and his colleagues in 1974, several other investigators have confirmed the efficacy of the treatment, which is reported to be effective in over 90% of patients with generalised plaque psoriasis. More recently PUVA therapy has been successfully applied in the treatment of mycosis fungoides (an uncommon malignant lymphoma that appears to originate in the skin) and atopic dermatitis (a common genetic form of eczema).

6.3.2 UV-A dosimetry in PUVA

The type of instrument used for determination of UV-A irradiance in treatment cubicles is normally a UV-A detector, the characteristics and performance of which have been described in § 4.5.2. However, as a biological monitor these devices are limited, in that the ideal UV-A detector in photochemotherapy would be an instrument whose spectral response matched the therapeutic action spectrum of the treatment, and which had an angular response weighted according to a cosine function with a wide angle of view suitable for use at short distances from extended arrays of fluorescent lamps. It is not yet possible to design such a detector, since the data relating to the therapeutic effectiveness of each wavelength in causing regression of the disease still remain uncertain. One end-point which has been considered is the erythema action spectrum of 8-MOP, but even in this field there is only limited agreement between workers. Nakayama *et al* (1974) found a broad spectrum for erythema in guinea-pig skin after 8-MOP in the range 320–380 nm with a maximum at 330 nm. Similar results were found by Owens *et al* (1968), whereas both Buck *et al* (1960) and Pathak (1961) found the same range for humans, but with a maximum at 360 nm. The latter of the two papers also showed essentially the same results for guinea-pig skin. It should also be pointed out that the spectra obtained by both Buck *et al* (1960) and Pathak (1961) were based on only small samples, i.e. three subjects in each study; and that, furthermore, these action spectra relate to the ability of different wavelengths to evoke an erythema response, which may bear no relationship to the ability to cause clearing of psoriatic lesions.

Notwithstanding these theoretical considerations, a recent survey (Diffey *et al* 1980) of the performance of commercial UV-A detectors in clinical use showed wide variations in accuracy, which may partly account for the apparent large differences in the total UV dose which has been reported as necessary to clear psoriatic lesions.

Since the topology of a human subject does not permit uniform irradiation, it is strictly incorrect to speak of a single treatment radiant exposure. The relative distribution of UV-A exposure on the surface of

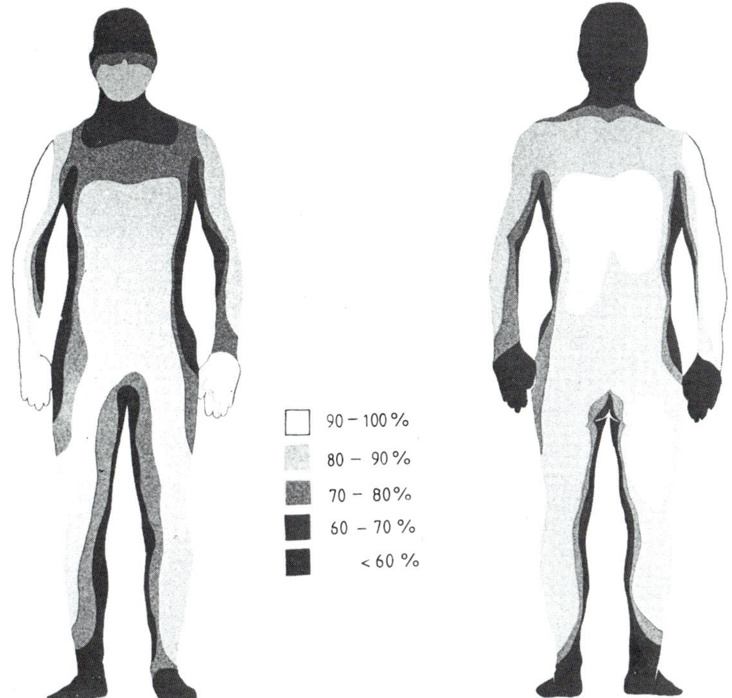

Figure 6.4 The relative distribution of UV-A exposure on the surface of a manikin resulting from whole-body irradiation in a step-in cubicle (from Diffey *et al* 1978).

a manikin resulting from whole-body irradiation in a step-in cubicle containing 62 fluorescent lamps is illustrated in figure 6.4. The measurements were made by attaching 65 UV-A film badges to the surface of an unclothed manikin (Diffey *et al* 1978). A large fraction of the body surface area receives more than 70% of the maximum exposure, although areas such as the axillae and groin receive a smaller fraction, as expected.

6.3.3 Risks of PUVA treatment

The short-term side effects that may occur during PUVA treatment are erythema, and possibly pruritus, due to UV-A overexposure, and nausea after ingestion of the drug, particularly with doses higher than 50 mg.

The possible long-term effects of the treatment include premature skin ageing, cutaneous carcinoma and cataract induction. The results of animal experiments suggest that oral administration of psoralens does not augment the carcinogenic effect of ultraviolet radiation to the same degree as psoralens administered topically or intraperitoneally. Also, psoralens and sunlight exposure have been used to treat pigment disorders such as vitiligo for 25 years and as yet there have been no reports of skin cancer in these patients. However a new compound, 3-carbethoxypsoralen, has recently been described (Dubertret *et al* 1979) which exhibits the same therapeutic effectiveness as 8-MOP when used in conjunction with UV-A but which appears to be far less mutagenic and carcinogenic.

Another potential drawback of long-term therapy associated with present PUVA treatment is the possibility of producing cataracts; eye damage has been produced in guinea pigs who were administered oral 8-methoxypsoralen and whose eyes were irradiated with monochromatic radiation from 300–390 nm in steps of 10 nm (Freeman and Troll 1969). There was evidence of ocular injury at 72 h post-irradiation at all wavelengths less than 380 nm, with maximum photosensitivity occurring between 320 and 340 nm. Consequently eye protection is provided during patient treatment by using goggles which are opaque to UVR.

Solar UV-A irradiance on cloudless days can be as high as 50 $W m^{-2}$, a value which is comparable with that encountered in treatment units. Since most of the UV-A that enters the pupil is absorbed by the crystalline lens of the eye (Boettner and Wolter 1962), and since free 8-MOP can be detected in human lenses for at least 12 h following oral ingestion (Lerman *et al* 1980) it is desirable that patients should wear suitable eye protection for the remainder of the day, to reduce the ingress of UV through the pupil to insignificant levels. A discussion of some of the protective eyewear that is available is given in § 7.5.3.2.

6.4 Phototherapy for Neonatal Jaundice

Neonatal jaundice, or hyperbilirubinaemia, is a common disorder found in about 10–20% of newborn babies. Hyperbilirubinaemia is an excess of the reddish-coloured bile pigment bilirubin (a decomposition product of haemoglobin) in the serum and is usually described as existing when the serum bilirubin concentration is higher than 15 mg per 100 ml of serum. If left untreated the condition may lead to permanent brain damage. Before 1958 the standard treatment was to carry out a tedious and hazardous exchange transfusion. In that year, however, Cremer and his colleagues showed that irradiation of jaundiced babies with blue light led to a fall in the serum bilirubin level. The favourable results obtained by phototherapy for neonatal jaundice have since been confirmed by several workers and phototherapy is now the treatment of choice by many paediatricians.

6.4.1 Principles of action

Bilirubin is a yellow compound and consequently strongly absorbs blue light, particularly in the wavelength region 400–480 nm. The action spectrum for the decomposition of bilirubin *in vitro* is shown in figure 6.5 and closely approximates the shape of the absorption spectrum. The mechanism of phototherapy *in vivo*, however, is obscure. Following irradiation of jaundiced babies with blue light two effects occur; the exposed skin becomes bleached and the concentration of bilirubin in the serum falls. The effects result from conversion of bilirubin to unidentified compounds which are more readily excreted, and stimulation of the hepatic excretion of unconjugated bilirubin.

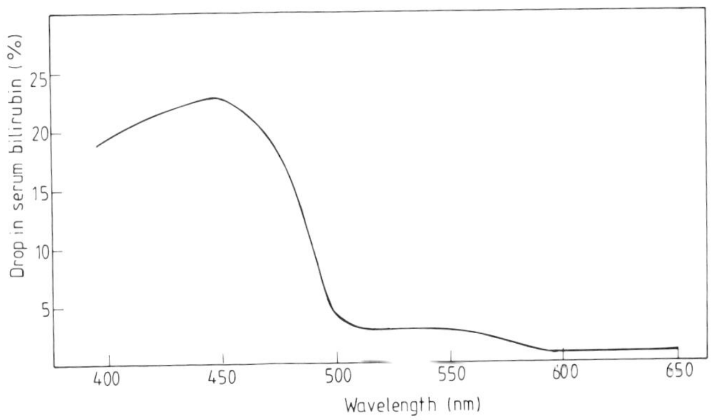

Figure 6.5 The action spectrum for the decomposition of serum bilirubin (from Cremer *et al* 1958).

6.4.2 Physical aspects

The lamps used in phototherapy irradiation units are invariably fluorescent tubes. Lamps emitting a broad spectral distribution from about 330–750 nm ('daylight' lamp) have been widely used, although a 'blue' lamp has been developed with its emission spectrum chiefly in the wavelength region 400–500 nm (e.g. the Philips 03T lamp). It is essential that a suitable UV absorbing material, such as Perspex VA acrylic plastic, be placed between the lamps and the baby to remove radiation with wavelengths less than about 380 nm.

The irradiance at the babies' skin depends, of course, on the design of the luminaire. An irradiance of around 20 $W m^{-2}$ in the spectral range 400–480 nm is typical at a distance of 450 mm from a unit incorporating four (20 W) blue fluorescent lamps, whilst a unit incorporating 10 (20 W) daylight fluorescent lamps only results in an irradiance of around 5 $W m^{-2}$ in the same spectral range and at the same distance.

6.4.3 Clinical aspects

The decision to treat a jaundiced baby with phototherapy is not automatic and needs careful consideration by the physician responsible for the care of the infant. A major factor to be considered is the immediate risk of alternative approaches for lowering serum bilirubin concentration to prevent damage to the central nervous system from hyperbilirubinaemia.

Following the decision to treat the baby with phototherapy, he is placed in a nursery cot, or even a purpose-built irradiation cot, with the lamps something like 400–800 mm above the baby. The baby's eyes should be closed and covered with a bandage during treatment to prevent exposure to light. The treatment schedule can vary but a regimen of six-hours-on, two-hours-off, has been widely used. Serum bilirubin levels should be assayed every 8–12 h to monitor the progress of the phototherapy, which may last from 1–6 d, depending upon the severity of the condition.

If the baby is irradiated in an open cot, or bassinet, the lamps should be adequately shielded to protect the infant from both UVR of wavelengths less than 380 nm, and broken glass should the lamp envelope implode. Also, units which incorporate the blue fluorescent lamps should include additionally at least one daylight lamp, since blue light may make it difficult for nursery personnel to detect cyanosis (bluish complexion from lack of oxygen in the blood circulating through the skin).

6.5 Relief of Pruritus by Phototherapy

Pruritus (itching) is a distressing feature of several unrelated clinical conditions. In two such conditions, primary biliary cirrhosis, and uraemia experienced by patients on chronic haemodialysis, a short course of phototherapy has been reported to alleviate itching.

In a pilot study involving six patients with primary biliary cirrhosis, daily irradiation of the whole body for 30–60 s with a medium-pressure mercury arc lamp relieved itching in five patients within one week of commencing exposure to UVR (Hanid and Levi 1980).

A larger study involving 18 patients with chronic renal failure requiring haemodialysis yielded similar encouraging results (Gilchrest *et al* 1977). All the patients had had pruritus for at least two months which was unresponsive to routine oral and topical medications. It was severe enough to disturb sleep and interfere with normal daytime activities. In this study ten of the patients were irradiated in a treatment cubicle containing 72 UV-B fluorescent sunlamps whilst the remaining eight patients were given phototherapy in a PUVA treatment cubicle incorporating 64 UV-A fluorescent lamps. The patients receiving UV-B radiation were given an initial dose equivalent to about 75% of the estimated minimal erythema dose (MED) and each subsequent treatment was lengthened by 25% of the MED. The treatment times of the patients in the UV-A group were matched to those in the UV-B group and, because of the higher irradiance from the UV-A lamps, resulted in higher doses. All patients received eight exposures to the whole body over a four-week period. At the end of this period, nine of the ten patients in the UV-B group reported a significant improvement in their pruritus as opposed to two of the eight patients in the UV-A group.

In both of these studies it would seem that UV-B is the effective waveband in relieving itching. Although the response mechanism is not known, it may be that its action is a local one on an 'itch receptor' in the skin. The encouraging results obtained with phototherapy suggest that it may be worth pursuing in other situations where pruritus is a troublesome symptom.

6.6 Photosensitivity Investigations

The accurate diagnosis of a suspected photosensitive patient demands above all a clear and detailed history. If the diagnosis still remains in doubt it may be worthwhile to carry out photobiological investigations using a solar simulator or an irradiation monochromator.

The details of the patient's history are very much the province of the clinical dermatologist, but some of the more important points may be worth considering here.

(1) The age of onset may be important in genetic disorders.

(2) The season of the year that the symptoms occur may give some guide to the wavelengths responsible. Patients who reside in the United Kingdom and only present with photosensitive symptoms in the middle of summer will probably be reacting to the UV-B region, since the irradiance in this waveband is about one hundred times higher in summer than in winter. Where the patient is photosensitive all the year round, the causative wavelengths are likely to be in the UV-A and visible regions, which show much less seasonal variations in irradiance than the UV-B region.

(3) Lesions usually occur only on those parts of the body exposed to sunlight. However in some photodermatoses, for example actinic reticuloid, lesions may also appear on clothed areas.

(4) The subjective sensations experienced by the patient in sunlight may be just as important as the appearance of erythema or morphological lesions. For example, a burning or tingling sensation is often a feature of erythropoietic protoporphyria.

(5) The time between exposure to light and the appearance of the lesion may sometimes be a helpful guide to diagnosis. The development of a weal either during or soon after irradiation is a classical feature associated with solar urticaria.

(6) The morphology of the lesion may help to establish a firm diagnosis.

(7) The occupation of the patient may give some clue to the cause of the photodermatosis. People working with known photosensitisers, such as tar or some pharmaceuticals, may have their skin contaminated. Welders using electric arcs without due regard for adequate safety precautions may be subject to intense UV-B and UV-C irradiation. Publicans may suffer an occupational hazard for alcoholism, which is sometimes associated with porphyria cutanea tarda.

(8) Cosmetic preparations may be responsible for the photosensitivity. Berloque dermatitis due to 5-methoxypsoralen contained in bergamot oil, a constituent of many perfumes, is the classic example in this category.

When a photodermatosis is suspected from the patient's history and clinical examination, it is desirable to proceed to photobiological investigations if irradiation facilities are available. The object of phototesting is twofold: to reproduce the disease so as to confirm the diagnosis; and to ascertain the action spectrum, so that suitable preventative measures can be taken. Simple testing in broad spectral regions can be performed with mercury arc lamps, or more preferably with the xenon arc lamp, in conjunction with optical filters. The xenon arc lamp has the advantage that its spectral power distribution is similar to terrestrial radiation and so is a more physiologically-suited source for studying diseases induced by sunlight. For this reason it is often referred to as a solar simulator (*see* § 2.3.5.1). The solar simulator may indicate the broad spectral regions to which the patient is responsive, e.g. UV-B, UV-A or visible, but is not suited to action spectra studies. For these studies an irradiation monochromator is required and careful investigations over the past 20 years have led to the clearer delineation of photodermatological syndromes and the characterisation of 'new' diseases.

6.6.1 Phototesting with an irradiation monochromator

The performance of irradiation monochromators has been discussed fully in Chapter 3 and so it will be assumed that the instrument is optimally aligned and properly calibrated. This section will briefly mention some of the practical aspects concerned with investigating the patient.

(1) The position of the patient during irradiation is not critical, so long as he remains still. It is usual for the patient to sit up with his back against the exit port of the monochromator. However, the recent availability of relatively cheap, liquid-filled, light guides, which transmit UVR at wavelengths down to 250 nm, has resulted in much greater flexibility for both the patient and operator. Figure 6.6 shows a patient being irradiated in this manner, with the light guide optically coupled to the exit slit of the monochromator by a quartz doublet lens. The light guide is supported on a flexible arm and so allows the patient to relax in a prone position during the investigation, which may take an hour or more.

(2) The dose range and increment must be such as to demonstrate the desired response. Historical practice has favoured the threshold response, or minimal erythema dose, as a measure of erythemal reactivity. If this is the response required then it should lie somewhere in the middle of a dose range. A given dose range is more economically covered by a geometrical series of dose increments rather than by an arithmetical series. Dose increments based on a ratio of $2^{1/2}$ have been used by some workers; this geometrical series is equivalent to doubling alternate doses.

(3) The anatomical site normally chosen for irradiation is the back,

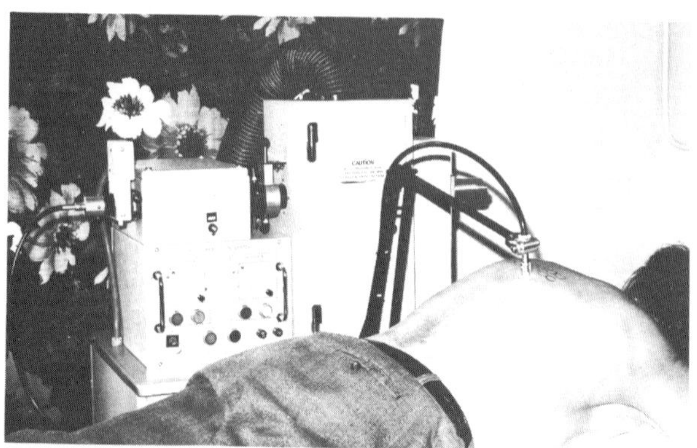

Figure 6.6 A patient being investigated for suspected photosensitivity with an irradiation monochromator. Note the liquid-filled light guide which is used to conduct the radiation from the exit port of the monochromator to the patient's skin.

since it combines a large surface area with reasonably uniform sensitivity to UVR. The mid two-thirds of the volar aspect of the forearm is reasonably uniform, but the photosensitivity at the wrist is much less and at the cubital fossa it may be higher.

(4) The results of irradiation are normally appraised visually at 24 h after exposure. However, if the patient is admitted to hospital for phototesting it may be possible, and also worthwhile, to assess the reactions both earlier and later. It is usual to rank the degree of reactions using an arbitrary scale such as 0, ±, +, ++, etc. More quantitative methods employing colour charts, optical filters and reflectance spectrometry have been used, but in most centres visual inspection is the method of choice. The recording of immediate responses is also important, together with any morphological changes and subjective sensations.

It would be imagined that a photodermatosis can be reproduced by exposing the patient's skin to an artificial source that produces the same wavelengths as those in sunlight which initiate the disease. In practice this procedure is not always rewarding, although it is not clear why laboratory photobiological studies sometimes fail to produce the expected response. Presumably variables such as irradiance, radiant exposure, size and anatomical location of irradiated skin, and synergism between wavelengths play some role, as may psychological factors and cyclic responses.

6.6.2 Photopatch testing

When the photodermatosis is suspected as a result of cutaneous contact with some photosensitiser, it is desirable to carry out so-called photopatch testing to try to reproduce the lesion. Techniques may vary somewhat, but essentially the procedure is as follows. The suspected agent is applied in duplicate sites on areas of skin not usually exposed to light (e.g. the lumbar region of the back) on a patch-test unit. A common patch-test unit used in the UK is the Al-Test, which consists of a round piece of filter paper, 10 mm in diameter, fastened centrally to a $25 \times 25\ mm^2$ impermeable sheet of aluminium foil coated with polythene. Forty-eight hours later one of the two patch test sites is uncovered and exposed to UV-A radiation. The sources used for UV-A irradiation in photopatch testing are usually either a bank of four fluorescent 'blacklight' lamps or a Kromayer lamp with a suitable glass filter (e.g. Schott WG345) to remove the UV-B and UV-C radiation. The radiant exposure should depend upon many factors such as the penetration of the test material into the skin and its quantum yield, which is related to the efficiency of the radiation in producing photoproducts. In clinical dermatology this information is generally unknown and so the radiant exposure is usually empirical. Experience has shown that many photoallergic reactions can be produced with doses at less than $10^4\ J\,m^{-2}$ of UV-A.

A further 48 h later both test sites are uncovered and the reactions assessed. If the irradiated site is positive and the non-irradiated site is negative then contact photoallergy can be diagnosed. If both sites show equal reactions the diagnosis is contact allergy alone. But if both sites are positive with a more severe reaction on the irradiated site, then the diagnosis is contact photoallergy and contact allergy.

6.6.3 Treatment of photosensitivity

When the cause of the photosensitivity is some exogeneous photosensitiser which has been identified by photopatch testing, the treatment is simply to eliminate cutaneous contact with the substance, if possible. This may involve the trivial solution of using another brand of perfume, or perhaps the more serious decision of changing occupation. However, when the photosensitivity is a result of some idiopathic photodermatosis, suitable treatment is not so readily forthcoming.

General advice given to photosensitive patients includes the avoidance of sunlight wherever possible and the wearing of protective clothing and sunscreen agents where this is not possible. Although high absorption of the UV-B waveband is readily achievable, there is no completely satisfactory sunscreen that absorbs through the UV-A and into the blue region of the visible spectrum. It is common practice for manufacturers of sunscreens to quote a 'protection factor' associated with their product and for photodermatological applications a protection factor of 10 or more is often desirable.

There is not yet available a systemic drug which is universally accepted as a satisfactory photoprotectant. The drugs mepacrine and chloroquine were fashionable at one time in treating polymorphic light eruption but are now out of favour with many dermatologists because of their adverse side effects. Successful management of this photodermatosis has been achieved in some patients by subjecting them to a short course of PUVA therapy in the spring so that the melanin pigmentation which develops can act as a protectant against the summer sun.

It has been reported (Mathews-Roth *et al* 1974) that oral beta-carotene is an effective systemic photoprotectant in patieints with erythropoietic protoporphyria, a disease which often results in photosensitivity throughout the UV-A region and visible spectrum. Not all investigators, however, have shown the same enthusiasm for the treatment (Magnus 1976); nevertheless the success achieved with this drug has provided impetus in the search for other oral sunscreens.

6.7 Luminescence Techniques in Diagnosis

The ultraviolet irradiation of many substances results in the excitation of one or more electrons in each molecule from the ground state to a higher energy state. The subsequent electron transition back to the ground state must be accompanied by the dissipation of energy, which may be as heat by interactions with the vibrating atoms in the substance, or by the emission of a photon of light of a wavelength greater than the exciting radiation. The latter process is termed luminescence. If the substance emits light simultaneously with its excitation the process is called fluorescence; if the substance continues to emit light for longer than 1 μs after the exciting radiation is switched off, then the process is termed phosphorescence.

Luminescence techniques are used for diagnosis in dermatology and dentistry. In both disciplines the exciting source is usually a Wood's lamp (*see* § 2.3.3.4); this is essentially a source of monochromatic 365 nm radiation which is often referred to as 'Wood's light'.

6.7.1 Dermatological applications

The Wood's lamp, illustrated in figure 6.7, has been used for many years by dermatologists. Some of the disorders which it is used to diagnose include the following.

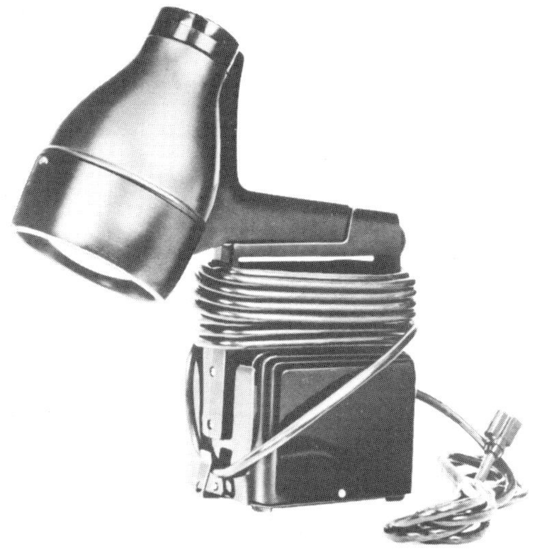

Figure 6.7 A Wood's lamp used for diagnosis. (Courtesy of Ultraviolet Products, Inc, San Gabriel, USA).

(1) Tinea capitis (ringworm)—this is a fungal infection of the scalp. Hairs which are infected with the fungi microsporon audouini or microsporon canis will fluoresce with a bright blue-green under Wood's light. The diagnosis can be confirmed by removing the fluorescent hairs for direct microscopic examination and culture.

(2) Erythrasma—a superficial bacterial infection of the skin, usually between two surfaces of skin that rub together (intertriginous areas), such as the groin or toe-webs. Erythrasma produces scaling and cracking and may be accompanied by pruritus (itching). The responsible organism (corynebacterium minutissimum) produces a porphyrin that fluoresces a bright coral-red colour on irradiation with a Wood's lamp.

(3) Porphyria cutanea tarda (PCT)—a member of the porphyria family of diseases (*see* § 5.4.2.1) often associated with alcoholism in middle-aged men. In PCT there is an excessive urinary excretion of uroporphyrin

which fluoresces with a pink or red colour on excitation with UV-A. The quantity of uroporyphyrin in freshly voided urine in severe PCT may be high enough for visible fluorescence without treatment, although often fluorescence is quenched. In such cases it is necessary to acidify the urine and to extract the porphyrin into amyl alcohol in which porphyrins fluoresce freely.

(4) Infection of burn wounds—the most common organism causing infection of burn wounds is pseudomonas aeruginosa. The onset of pseudomonas burn sepsis is often insidious. The organism is notoriously resistant to many anti-bacterial agents and delayed diagnosis of infection can greatly increase the risk of mortality. However, early recognition of the organism is possible since it produces the bacterial pigment fluoresencein which fluoresces with a yellow-green colour under Wood's light.

6.7.2 Dental applications

Irradiation of the oral cavity with a Wood's lamp will produce fluorescence which may prove useful in the diagnosis of various dental disorders, such as early dental caries (tooth decay); the incorporation of tetracycline into teeth; dental plaque (a polysaccharide that adheres to the tooth surface); and calculus (a chalky deposit on the teeth mainly precipitated from saliva).

Normal teeth fluoresce with a light blue colour. The application of the dye fluorescein (not to be confused with the bacterial pigment mentioned in the previous section) to the teeth followed by irradiation with UV-A more readily allows plaque to be visualised than with visible light. The presence of calculus on the teeth will result in a yelloworange fluorescence under UV-A illumination.

The administration of the antibiotic tetracycline can result in its incoporation into the tooth structure. Such teeth have a yellowish-brown discolouration in visible light but fluoresce with an intense yellow when exposed to Wood's light.

6.8 Non-clinical Applications of Ultraviolet Radiation

Apart from its role in the diagnosis and treatment of disease, UVR is also employed in several non-clinical situations in medicine. In this section some of these applications will be discussed briefly.

6.8.1 Polymerisation of dental resins

The restoration of pits and fissures in both deciduous and permanent teeth is often accomplished by using an adhesive resin polymerised with UV-A. The resin is applied to the surfaces to be treated with a fine brush and is hardened by exposure to the UV-A radiation from a Wood's lamp for 30 s or so. The restoration of teeth by resinous sealants is not only more aesthetically acceptable to patients than repair using conventional materials, but offers greater protection against tooth decay at the sites of pits and fissures.

6.8.2 Sterilisation

The lethal effect of UV-C radiation on bacteria has been known for about 100 years. A typical action spectrum for the bactericidal effect of UVR is shown in figure 6.8 and exhibits a peak in the range 260–270 nm. This action spectrum is similar to the absorption spectrum of nucleic acids and for this reason the important molecule deoxyribonucleic acid (DNA) is thought to be the main target.

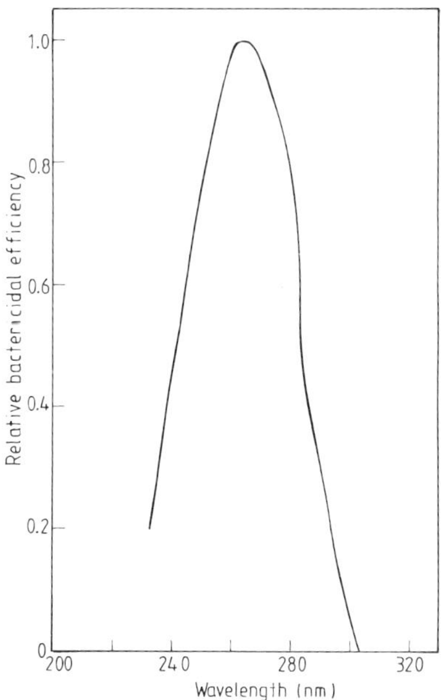

Figure 6.8 A typical action spectrum for the bactericidal effect of ultraviolet radiation.

The low-pressure mercury discharge lamp ('germicidal lamp') has a strong spectral emission at a wavelength of 254 nm (*see* figure 2.6), close to the peak of the action spectrum, and consequently is a very efficient bactericidal agent. The germicidal lamp has been incorporated into tissue culture cabinets and bacteriological handling hoods for the sterilisation of clinical and laboratory instruments. The success of these applications depends upon the surfaces being initially clean and free from films which would act to absorb the radiation and so reduce its bactericidal effect.

Germicidal lamps have also been installed in rooms such as operating theatres, microbiological laboratories and wards to disinfect the air. The design of such installations requires careful thought so that the amount of radiation received by persons within the room will not result in undesirable effects such as erythema or conjunctivitis. Alternatively, automatic switching gear can be linked to the entry door so that the lamps are only operational when there are no personnel in the room.

6.8.3 Inspection of intensifying screens

Intensifying screens are commonly used in radiography to provide a method of converting x-rays to ultraviolet and visible photons, to which photographic emulsion is responsive, and so obtaining, after processing, a comparable degree of blackening for a smaller exposure. The intensifying screens commonly used in medical radiography consist of a thin layer of calcium tungstate crystals suspended in a suitable binder and coated onto a semi-flexible support of plastic or card. Between the fluorescent layer and the support there is sometimes a reflecting layer of white pigment. The surface of the fluorescent layer is protected by an extremely thin, waterproof, transparent coating (supercoat).

In order to ensure optimum performance from intensifying screens it is important to inspect them carefully at regular intervals so that possible marks or defects in the supercoat may be observed. Efficient visual inspection of intensifying screens is best achieved under UV-C illumination. An apparatus which has been designed for this purpose is shown in figure 6.9. It consists of an 8 W germicidal lamp supported on a frame and shielded by a blue Perspex (type 703) hood. When the undamaged intensifying screen is irradiated with the lamp, a faint blue hue is observed due to reflection of the lines at 405 nm and 436 nm present in the emission spectrum. The 254 nm line which would normally excite the calcium tungstate fluorescent layer is partially reflected and partially absorbed completely by the supercoat. However, if the screen

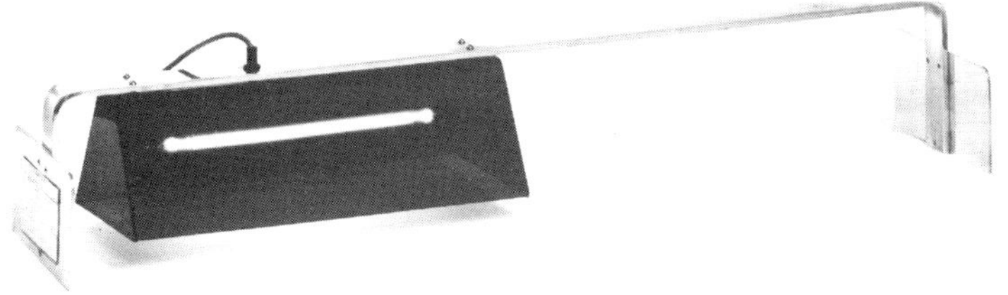

Figure 6.9 An apparatus for the inspection of intensifying screens used in radiography (from Diffey and Mallion 1978).

is scratched the supercoat is removed and exposes the fluorescent layer. The 254 nm radiation is now able to excite the calcium tungstate layer, which fluoresces with a bright blue colour. The spectral transmission properties of the blue Perspex hood are such that it will efficiently transmit the blue fluorescent radiation from the calcium tungstate whilst at the same time absorbing any ambient white light which may be reflected from the intensifying screen, together with complete absorption of reflected 254 nm radiation. This results in a high efficiency for visual detection of flaws in the supercoat coupled with complete safety from exposure to the ultraviolet radiation emitted by the lamp. Flaws in the supercoat which are of the order of 0.02 mm in width have been readily visualised with the apparatus.

7 Personal Exposure to Ultraviolet Radiation

It is well established that exposure to ultraviolet radiation can have both beneficial and detrimental effects on humans.

Although only relatively low doses of UVR are required to form measurable levels of vitamin D in the skin, people deprived of UVR are more liable to develop osteomalacia, particularly when there is impaired utilisation or dietary insufficiency of vitamin D. Groups which have been found to show low levels of vitamin D associated with chronic under-exposure to UVR are the elderly, submariners and Asiatic imigrants.

On the other hand, excessive repeated exposure to UVR is well known to induce both skin cancer and ageing effects. Also the increasing use of drugs which have photosensitivity side effects (e.g. phenothiazines, nalidixic acid and certain tetracyclines), have made a greater percentage of the population more liable to show abnormal sensitivity to UVR.

At present, environmental conservationists are becoming increasingly concerned that changes in the atmospheric ozone mantle may be induced by both high flying supersonic aircraft and by the build up of freons and related compounds. Should significant changes occur in the depth of the ozone layer, then it can be expected that the amount of UVR reaching the Earth's surface will be altered. Coupled with this is the steady increase in the number of artificial ultraviolet sources available for medical, industrial, military and cosmetic use, which has necessitated the introduction of safety standards for UV exposure.

This chapter reports on some recent studies of personal exposure to environmental UVR and current standards associated with occupational exposure to UVR.

7.1 Description of a Personal UVR Dosimeter

A recent report by the World Health Organization (WHO 1979) on environmental health criteria for ultraviolet radiation has recommended that certain studies be carried out to obtain the information required both for the adequate evaluation of health risks and for the establishment of appropriate protective measures and guidelines. The report stresses that population studies using personal monitoring devices for UV-B radiation are needed to determine the fraction of the daily natural UV dose received by persons at risk either from UVR deficiency or excess, or from occupational exposure, and concludes that the development of personal UVR monitoring devices is of the utmost priority.

Natural UVR is generally measured with solid state detectors, often used in conjunction with optical filters. In particular the Robertson–Berger meter, which measures those wavelengths in the global spectrum less than 320 nm, has been used to monitor natural UVR continuously at several sites throughout the world. A different, yet complimentary, approach is the use of various photosensitive films as UVR dosimeters. The principle is to relate the degree of deterioration of the films, usually in terms of changes in their optical properties, to the incident UVR dose. The principal advantages of the film dosimeter are that it provides a simple means of integrating UVR exposure continuously and that it allows numerous sites, inaccessible to bulky and expensive instrumentation, to be compared simultaneously.

In 1976, Davis and his colleagues reported the potential of the polymer film, polysulphone, as a personal UVR dosimeter. The basis of the method is that when polysulphone film is exposed to UVR at wavelengths less than 330 nm, the UV absorption of the film increases. The increase in absorbance measured at a wavelength of 330 nm is proportional to UV dose, and so the film readily lends itself to application as a UV dosimeter. In practice the film, 40 μm thick, is mounted in cardboard photographic holders with a central aperture of 12 × 16 mm (*see* figure 7.1), and worn

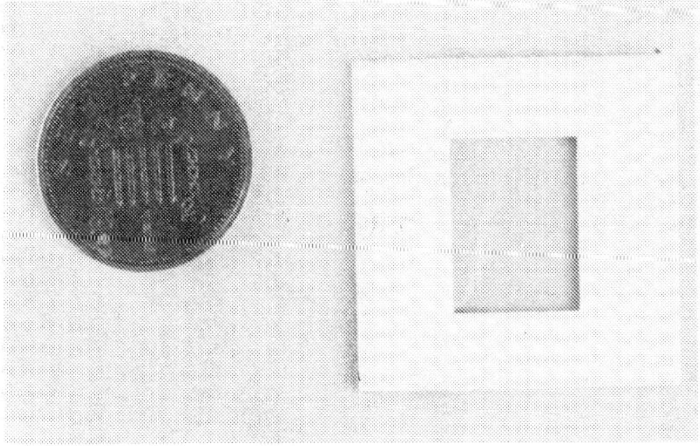

Figure 7.1 A polysulphone film badge.

by subjects much as photographic film badges are worn as ionising radiation monitors.

The principal limitation of the polysulphone film in this form has been that its sensitivity extends to wavelengths up to 330 nm, whereas the biological effectiveness of UVR is largely confined to wavelengths less than about 315 nm. This small difference in spectral response can lead to significant errors in estimates of the biologically-effective UV-B (*see* § 4.5.1) when the film is used to monitor natural UVR, due to the rapid increase in spectral irradiance of the solar spectrum between 315 and 330 nm. Nevertheless it is possible to relate polysulphone response to an erythemally-effective UV-B radiant exposure by carrying out correction calculations analagous to equations 4.8 and 4.9. To circumvent this limitation a much thinner polysulphone film (1 μm thick) mounted on a cellophane substrate has recently been developed (Davis *et al* 1981).

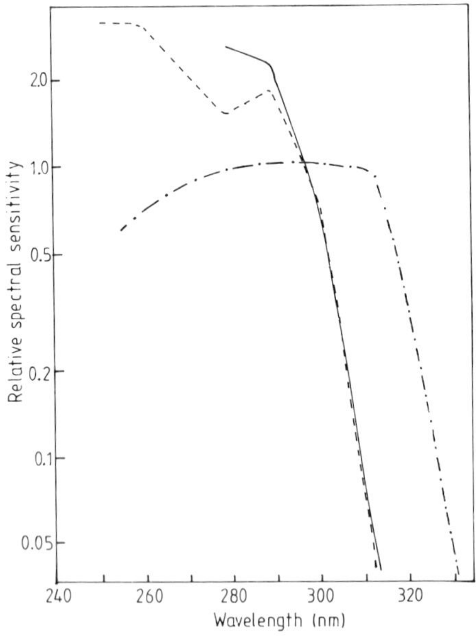

Figure 7.2 The spectral response of polysulphone film and the erythema action spectrum in normal human skin, normalised to unity at a wavelength of 297 nm: full curve, 1 μm thick polysulphone film mounted on a cellophane substrate (Davis *et al* 1981); chain curve, 40 μm thick polysulphone film (Davis *et al* 1976); and broken curve, erythema action spectrum (Mackenzie and Frain-Bell 1973).

The spectral sensitivity of the thinner film is shown in figure 7.2 and is compared with the 40 μm thick film, together with the erythema action spectrum in normal human skin. The agreement between the 1 μm thick polysulphone film mounted on a cellophane substrate and the erythema action spectrum is good in the wavelength region between 295 and 315 nm, which is important for monitoring devices designed for natural ultraviolet radiation.

Some of the applications of the 40 μm thick polysulphone film as a personal UVR dosimeter will be outlined in the next section.

7.2 Applications of Personal UVR Monitoring

7.2.1 Studies of UVR exposure to people in different environments

It is evident that the natural UVR exposure received by different individuals will depend not only upon the quality and quantity of the UV environment but also on the behaviour of the individuals concerned. It would be expected that outdoor workers, for example, would by and large receive much greater personal UVR doses than indoor workers. Nevertheless it is difficult to estimate from the recordings of stationary UV-B detectors the typical doses received by people under a variety of situations. It is, then, in the area of personal UVR dosimetry that polymer film badges have been most widely used.

In all of the studies to date the polymer film badges have been worn on the lapel site as this site is judged to receive approximately the same solar UVR dose as the hands and face. The results of various field studies (Challoner *et al* 1976; Leach *et al* 1978) are summarised in table 7.1.

Table 7.1 Representative personal erythemally-effective UVR doses received by different groups of people (adapted from Challoner *et al* 1976 and Leach *et al* 1978).

Group	Fraction of ambient dose received
Gardeners	0.10
Patients exposed to sunshine on balcony	0.10
Laboratory and office workers	0.03
Ward-fast patients	0.001

The effective erythemal dose at 297 nm is expressed as a fraction of the ambient dose available on an unshaded, horizontal surface, determined either by experimental measurement or by calculation using the model described in § 2.1.2. The doses are expressed in this manner since it has been found that the fraction of the ambient dose received is more or less independent of season and climatic conditions, whereas the absolute doses will vary by about two orders of magnitude from winter to summer. In London, for example, the ambient daily, erythemally-effective dose under clear day conditions is calculated to be about 1300 $\mathrm{J\,m^{-2}}$ in mid-summer and only 9 $\mathrm{J\,m^{-2}}$ in mid-winter.

The very low doses received by the ward-fast patients in table 7.1 is not surprising, since normal window glass has negligible transmission below 310 nm. This may help explain the high incidence of vitamin D deficiency in such patients; it is known that exposure to UVR in the range 290–310 nm is required for the photosynthesis of cholecalciferol.

Most indoor workers will receive their highest environmental UV-B exposure whilst on vacation. This is reflected in the results of carrying out personal UVR dosimetry measurements for the four different leisure pursuits of sun-seeking, skiing, sightseeing and sailing. These results are summarised in table 7.2, where by far the largest doses are received from sedentary occupations such as sunbathing. The fractions of ambient UVR received whilst sightseeing or sailing are not inconsistent with the fraction of 0.1 received by the outdoor workers in table 7.1. The fraction received whilst skiing is a little higher and may be due to increased UV-B reflected from the snow, the large amount of time spent in an upright posture, and the absence of shade from buildings, trees, sails, and so on.

All the groups in these studies showed relatively large standard deviations of the mean fraction of ambient dose received. This may have

Table 7.2 Representative personal erythemally-effective UVR doses received by people on vacation (Diffey *et al* 1982).

Pastime	Fraction of ambient dose received
Sunbathing on beach	0.75
Sitting by swimming pool	0.40
Skiing	0.22
Sightseeing	0.17
Sailing	0.14

been due to the position and plane in which the badge was worn, and to the behaviour of the individual with regard to posture, time spent in the sun, and so on.

7.2.2 UVR and drug photosensitivity of the skin

There are many oral drugs that appear to cause skin photosensitivity. The diagnosis of photosensitivity is often made clinically from the history presented by the patient. The dose of a therapeutic drug is normally known where a patient suffers an adverse photosensitive effect, but the radiant exposure of sunlight received is unknown. This factor is probably just as important as the drug and its dose in assessing diagnosis and in planning treatment and prevention. Personal UVR dosimetry may then be useful in this respect and the findings of one such investigation (Corbett *et al* 1978) are summarised below.

The study was carried out in groups of 5–6 institutionalised psychiatric patients on phenothiazine therapy. Chlorpromazine was the most commonly prescribed drug and commonly causes skin photosensitivity as an adverse side effect. The project was done in five separate hospitals, four in England, one in Eire. The medical and nursing staff recorded daily the hours that each of the patients under study spent out of doors in bright sunlight over July and August, 1976. They also recorded symptoms of photosensitivity on a special form provided; from this a simple numerical scoring system for the severity of photosensitive symptoms was derived which could be compared with UVR dose recorded by the polysulphone film badge.

On analysis of the results it was found that badge dose and the recorded hours as spent in direct sunlight had a stong positive correlation ($p < 0.001$). What was especially interesting was that the badge dose also correlated positively with the symptom score of the patients ($p < 0.001$), but that symptom score and hours outdoors did not correlate; this is plausible, for the time outdoors in our climate will include many periods of overcast weather. These results suggest that, given suitable situations, this method is a valid approach for collecting objective data where previously results were subjective and conclusions had to be tentative.

7.2.3 UVR and long-stay geriatric patients

One of the features of long-stay geriatric patients is the high incidence of osteomalacia coupled with very low levels of plasma-25-hydroxyvitamin D [25(OH)D]. Such levels are due to a combination of negligible exposure to sunlight, and poor absorption and dietary intake of vitamin D. Corless *et al* (1978) have examined the efficacy of artificial UVR in restoring plasma-25-(OH)D to normal in patients in long-stay geriatric wards in the following study.

Banks of eight UV-B fluorescent sunlamps, (Westinghouse FS20) which emit a spectrum extending from 270–380 nm peaking at 313 nm, (*see* figure 2.8) were suspended from the ceilings of the ward dayrooms and the patients were irradiated for 3 h each day. The patients were dressed so that the head and neck, forearms and hands, and legs below the knees were exposed (about 0.4 m^2 of skin) and each patient wore on her lapel a polysulphone film badge. The UV dose recorded by the film badge was expressed in terms of equivalent radiant exposure at the most effective wavelength for healing of rickets, namely 280 nm. In order to express the dose in this manner, allowance was made for the differences between the spectral power distribution of the Westinghouse sunlamp, the spectral response of 40 μm thick polysulphone film, and the action spectrum for antirachitic activity (*see* figure 5.6).

The results showed that supplementation of the ward lighting by UVR increased plasma-25(OH)D in the patients by an amount sufficient to bring the level in depleted subjects into the normal range. The UV dose rate required to achieve this increase is about 85 $J\,m^{-2}\,d^{-1}$; about 25–50% of the minimal erythema dose. However, the threshold limit value for occupational exposure to actinic radiation has been set at 30 $J\,m^{-2}$ per 8 h period of exposure (*see* §7.3). This is about one third of the required therapeutic dose, and so potential problems may arise with regard to the UV doses received by people such as nursing staff.

7.2.4 The anatomical distribution of sunlight

The simplicity of film dosimetry allows numerous sites to be compared simultaneously and this lends itself readily to measuring the anatomical distribution of sunlight. One purpose of this work was to look at the supposed correlation between sunlight exposure and the distribution of skin cancer on the body surface. The relative distribution of short-wave, natural UVR at ten sites on the surface of an unclothed manikin was measured using polysulphone film as the dosimeter (Diffey *et al* 1977).

The manikin was positioned in a normal upright posture with arms at the side on an unshaded lawn and rotated on a turntable at 0.5 rev min^{-1} for 2 h, one hour either side of solar noon on several different days during the summer of 1976, a period which proved to have large variations in cloud cover. The measurements were made at

Canterbury, England (latitude 51 °N, altitude 40 m above sea level). Since the change of solar altitude is negligible during one revolution of the manikin, its rotation at a constant velocity may be regarded as equivalent to the 'random' motion of a human subject outdoors.

If the dose on the vertex is taken at 100%, it was found that on approximately horizontal surfaces such as the top of the shoulders (epaulet region) and the dorsa of the feet, where there will be some shading from the rest of the body, the value is about 80% of the vertex. Approximately vertical planes on the body received about 60%, mostly UVR not directly from the sun. It was also observed that the relative dose at each site was approximately independent of cloud cover.

The results obtained may be used to give a qualitative indication of erythemal or carcinogenic UVR at different anatomical sites, since the anatomical distribution of the waveband 295–310 nm, which includes most of the normal sunburning wavelengths and presumably those causing skin cancer, will be very similar to that of 295–330 nm, which encompasses the action spectrum of the polysulphone film.

These measurements indicate that the hands receive roughly the same UVR dose as the face. This is in harmony with the clinical observation that the skin changes in the commoner idiopathic photodermatoses are mostly located on these regions. This is also in agreement with the distribution of squamous cell epitheliomas. *Per contra* the incidence of basal-cell epitheliomas on the face is about an order of magnitude higher than on the hands. This apparent discrepancy strongly suggests that sunlight is not the only factor in the aetiology of carcinoma of the skin, particularly basal-cell carcinomas, a conclusion which has been voiced by several workers.

Since more than 90% of basal cell carcinomas (BCC) occur on the head and neck, a further study was carried out during the summer of 1978 to measure in detail the distribution of global UVR on the face and to relate the findings to published data on the facial distribution of BCC (Diffey *et al* 1979).

In order to allow a sufficiently high degree of spatial resolution of measurement across the face, a large fibreglass model of a head was constructed with all linear dimensions increased by a factor of approximately three. Polysulphone film badges were located on 41 numbered sites on the head by means of elastic bands. This method of attachment of badges was simple, quick and reproducible, and allowed the badges to be as close to the 'skin' as possible (*see* figure 7.3).

The whole assembly was placed outdoors, with low buildings on two

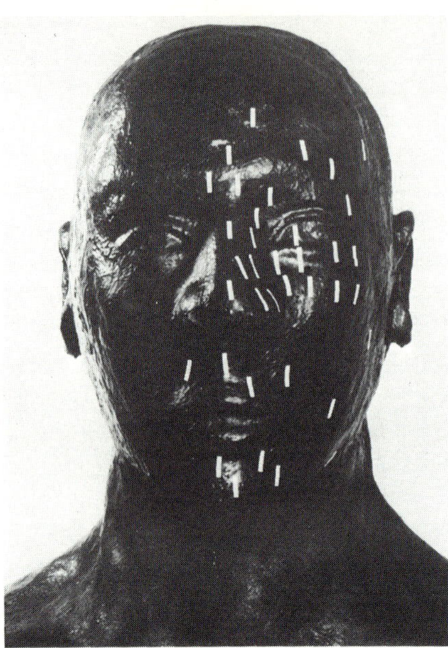

Figure 7.3 The fibreglass head showing the sites to which polysulphone film badges were attached. (Reprinted by permission from *Nature* **261** 169. Copyright © 1976 Macmillan Journals Limited.)

sides and open grass on the other two, and the head rotated for 3 h around solar noon each day for nine different days during August 1978.

The results indicated a 100-fold range of UV dose over the face, the vertex always being the site of maximum dose. It was evident that regions such as the orbits, philtrum, sublabial area, and submental area receive very little UVR. The results were correlated with the distribution of BCC in various cutaneous sites on the head given by Brodkin *et al* (1969). The distribution of tumours on the head and neck classified by these workers is illustrated in figure 7.4. A least squares fit of the logarithm of tumour density against the logarithm of UV dose as the dependent variable gave

$$\text{tumour density} \propto (\text{UV dose})^p, \qquad (7.1)$$

where $p = 1.71 \pm 0.33$, with a correlation coefficient of 0.69. Although the value obtained for the exponent, or 'biological amplification factor', is in substantial agreement with that derived from epidemiological studies

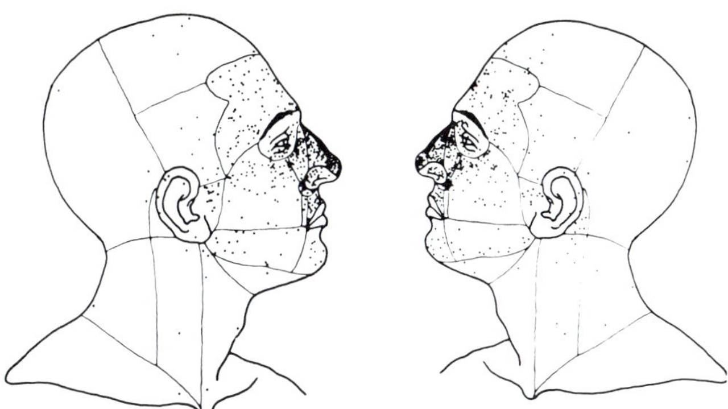

Figure 7.4 The distribution of basal cell carcinomas on the head and neck (from Brodkin *et al* 1969).

(*see* § 5.3.5.2), the poor correlation clearly questions the validity of the present comparison. The tumours were recorded at a different geographical location (New York: latitude 41 °N) from the measurements (Canterbury: latitude 51 °N) and their occurrence is presumably related to all-year-round sunlight exposure for many years. Furthermore, it is apparent that skin tumours originate in living cells in the viable layer of the epidermis, and so the tumour frequency would be expected to depend upon either the UV flux which reaches the critical cells or on products of UV damage to more superficial skin which reach the critical cells by diffusion, or both. Whatever the mechanism, the thickness of the stratum corneum could well be critically important, and there is no reason to suppose that the thickness of this layer is constant for all the sites chosen in the present comparison. Nevertheless, the results are compatible with the hypotheses that (a) human skin cancer incidence increases with environmental UVR exposure, and (b) sunlight is not the only factor in the aetiology of basal cell carcinomas of the face.

7.3 Occupational Ultraviolet Exposure Standards

At the present time there are no internationally agreed limits for occupational exposure to UVR. The most comprehensive occupational exposure standard for incoherent (non-laser) UV sources which has been published is that of the American Conference of Governmental

Industrial Hygienists. This standard has been endorsed by the National Institute for Occupational Safety and Health (NIOSH) in the United States and adopted as a voluntary standard in the United Kingdom by the Health and Safety Executive (HSE) and the National Radiological Protection Board (NRPB).

The exposure standard is considered separately for the UV-A region, and for the UV-B and UV-C regions, since most acute biological effects are initiated by wavelengths less than 315 nm.

7.3.1 UV-A exposure standard

For the spectral region 400–315 nm (UV-A), the total irradiance incident on unprotected eyes and skin for periods of greater than 1000 s should not exceed 10 $W\,m^{-2}$, and for exposure times of 1000 s or less than total radiant exposure of unprotected eyes and skin should not exceed $10^4\,J\,m^{-2}$.

7.3.2 UV-B and UV-C exposure standard

The exposure standard for the spectral region 315–200 nm (UV-B and UV-C) is based on an envelope action spectrum which combines the photokeratitis and skin erythema action spectra and which is defined as a smooth curve somewhat below the energies required for the development of observable effects. The standard, which applies to occupational exposure during an 8 h working day, is illustrated in figure 7.5 and shows maximum sensitivity at a wavelength of 270 nm and an exposure dose of 30 $J\,m^{-2}$. Maximum permissible exposures (MPEs) are also presented in table 7.3 together with the spectral effectiveness of the radiation relative to a wavelength of 270 nm. The MPE for monochromatic UVR sources in the wavelength region 315–200 nm can be determined directly from figure 7.5 or table 7.3. For broadband UVR sources, an effective irradiance, E_{eff}, is calculated by summing the contributions from all the spectral components of the source, each contribution being weighted by the relative spectral effectiveness, according to

$$E_{eff} = \sum E_s(\lambda)\, S(\lambda)\, \Delta\lambda, \tag{7.2}$$

where E_{eff} is effective irradiance relative to a monochromatic source at 270 nm ($W\,m^{-2}$); $E_s(\lambda)$ is the spectral irradiance at wavelength λ ($W\,m^{-2}\,nm^{-1}$); $S(\lambda)$ is the relative spectral effectiveness at wavelength λ; and $\Delta\lambda$ is the bandwidth employed in the measurement or calculation of $E_s(\lambda)$ (nm).

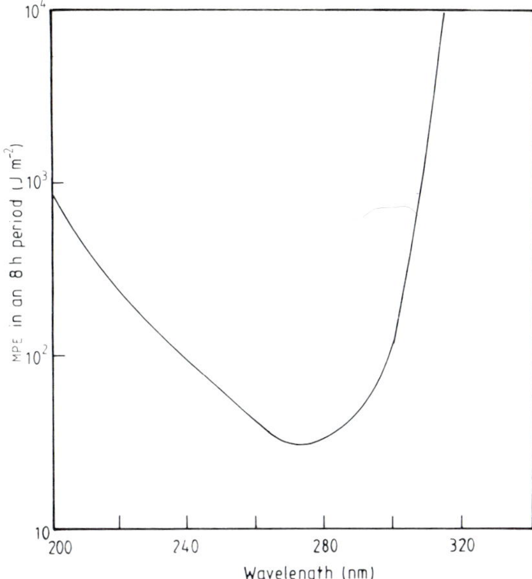

Figure 7.5 Envelope action spectrum used to define maximum permissible exposure (MPE) to ultraviolet radiation for an 8 h period (from NIOSH 1972).

Table 7.3 Maximum permissible exposuure (MPE) for eight-hour period (NRPB 1977).

Wavelength nm	MPE $J\,m^{-2}$	Relative spectral effectiveness, $S(\lambda)$
200	1000	0.03
210	400	0.075
220	250	0.12
230	160	0.19
240	100	0.30
250	70	0.43
254	60	0.5
260	46	0.65
270	30	1.0
280	34	0.88
290	47	0.64
300	100	0.30
305	500	0.06
310	2000	0.015
315	10000	0.003

The maximum permissible exposure time t_{max}, is then calculated as

$$t_{max} = 30(\mathrm{J\,m^{-2}})/E_{eff}(\mathrm{W\,m^{-2}})\ \mathrm{s}. \tag{7.3}$$

The method of summation described by equation (7.2) assumes that there are no synergistic or protective interactions between wavelengths, although it is unlikely that these assumptions are true.

For UVR sources which emit line spectra arranged in simple exposure geometries, it may be possible to assess the MPE by calculation. In most practical situations, however, recourse to measurement is probably necessary.

7.4 Instrumentation for Assessing UV Exposure Hazards

The experimental determination of a UV exposure hazard is necessary either when the spectral power distribution of the source is unknown, or when the geometry of the source makes calculation prohibitive.

The most fundamental method is to measure the spectral irradiance of the source, $E_s(\lambda)$ and to combine this data with the relative spectral effectiveness, $S(\lambda)$, in order to calculate an effective irradiance, E_{eff}, as given by equation (7.2). However this technique requires a spectroradiometer with high spectral resolution coupled with extremely good rejection of stray radiation, and probably demands a double monochromator. It is also necessary to calibrate the system against a standard lamp of known spectral irradiance, such as a deuterium arc or a tungsten–halogen lamp. In particular the uncertainties associated with the spectral irradiance from an incandescent source are highest at wavelengths below 300 nm due to lack of sufficient radiation.

Because of the severe experimental difficulties associated with absolute spectral radiometry, an assessment of the potential hazard from a UVR source is usually made through the use of a direct reading instrument whose spectral response has been designed to match the NIOSH 'hazard curve'. Such an instrument which is commercially available is the IL730A actinic radiometer (*see* figure 7.6), manufactured by International Light, Inc. This device incorporates a quartz wide angle diffuser, an interference filter, a blocking filter, and a 'solar blind' vacuum phototube as the detector. The published spectral response of a typical instrument is shown in figure 7.7. The spectral response of the instrument is an adequate match to the NIOSH curve in the wavelength range 250–300 nm, but the response at longer wavelengths may give cause for concern. The solar blind vacuum phototube can exhibit variations in its long wavelength response due to changes in the photoemissivity of the cathode with time and temperature. This can give rise to severe errors when trying to estimate the actinic hazard associated with sources which have a high UV-A component but whose spectral distribution in the actinic region extends only a short way below 315 nm. The most common example of such a source in medicine is probably the UV-A lamp used in photochemotherapy (*see* figure 2.9).

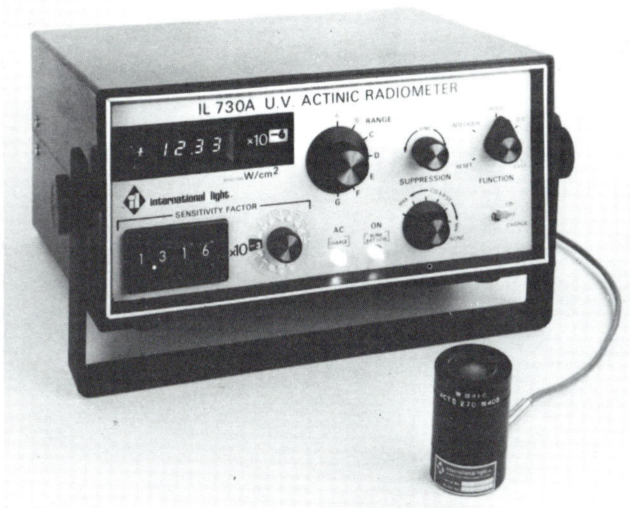

Figure 7.6 The IL730A actinic radiometer. (Courtesy of International Light Inc, Newburyport, Mass, USA.)

A survey of the levels of irradiance around three common sources of ultraviolet radiation found in physiotherapy departments has been carried out by the author using an IL730A actinic radiometer, and the results are summarised in table 7.4. The levels of UVR are quoted in terms of an effective irradiance in $W\,m^{-2}$ and so the MPE time (in seconds) is calculated by dividing this irradiance into the MPE for 270 nm radiation ($30\,J\,m^{-2}$). It is evident that a severe occupational exposure hazard exists in the direct beam of a Kromayer or Alpine lamp. Measurement of the effective irradiance in the vicinity of the beds used with the Alpine sunlamp and Theraktin UV bath indicated a MPE time of the order of

Table 7.4 Exposure hazard associated with three sources of ultraviolet radiation used in physiotherapy departments.

Irradiation unit	Lamp	Typical treatment distance	Typical treatment time	Effective irradiance ($W\,m^{-2}$) at treatment distance (MPE time in parentheses)
Kromayer lamp	medium-pressure mercury vapour arc in a quartz envelope	contact	2 s	240 (0.1 s)
Alpine sunlamp	medium-pressure mercury vapour arc in an envelope designed not to emit ozone-producing radiation	0.5 m	3 min	7 (4 s)
Theraktin ultraviolet bath	Four Westinghouse FS40 fluorescent sunlamps (1.22 m long)	0.5 m	5–30 min	0.4 (75 s)

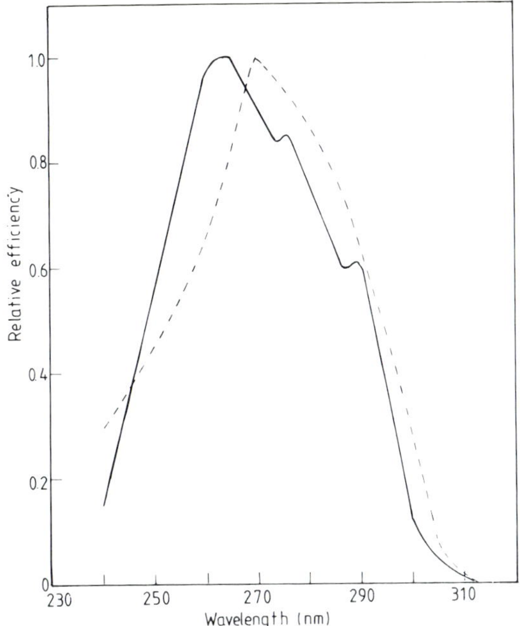

Figure 7.7 The published spectral response of the IL730A actinic radiometer (full curve) used in conjunction with a SEE 240 solar blind vacuum phototube and an ACTS 270 filter compared with the NIOSH relative spectral efficiency curve (broken curve).

10 min. Consequently it would be inadvisable for staff to remain in the immediate vicinity of the patient during treatment with these two units due to the presence of scattered and reflected radiation from the patient's skin, sheets and so on. In fact it is the custom in many physiotherapy departments for screens to be drawn around the patient and lamp during treatment and invariably the patient is issued UV opaque goggles.

7.5 Occupational Protection against Overexposure to UVR

Protection against overexposure to UVR may be achieved by a combination of administrative measures, engineering design and personal protection. It is desirable to place emphasis on administrative and engineering control measures so as to minimise the need for personal protection.

7.5.1 Administrative measures

7.5.1.1 Limitation of access. Only persons directly concerned with the work in hand should be permitted access to areas where there is equipment emitting UVR.

7.5.1.2 Hazard awareness. Persons working with UV equipment should be given adequate instruction as to the hazards associated with UVR. To this end 'local rules' could usefully be prepared and issued as appropriate.

7.5.1.3 Hazard warning signs and lights. Indication of the presence of a potential UVR hazard can be given by the judicious use of warning signs and lights should be used to show when the equipment is energised.

7.5.1.4 Distance and time as safety factors. As with ionising sources of radiation, the user should always bear in mind the protection afforded by maximising distance from the source and minimising exposure time. As a rule of thumb, at distances in excess of twice the greatest dimension of the source the intensity falls off according to the inverse square law, whereas at shorter distances the intensity falls off approximately linearly with distance. The exposure time should be such so as not to exceed the MPE time given by equation (7.3)

7.5.2 Engineering design

7.5.2.1 Containment of the radiation. Wherever it is reasonably practicable, the UVR should be kept within a sealed housing. If exposure takes place external to the source housing, as in patient irradiation, the radiation should be contained within a screened area by using, for example, dark cotton curtains. If observation of the UV source is required, then the viewing port should be made of a material with appropriate absorbing properties. Perspex VA acrylic sheet 6 mm thick is a convenient material for this purpose since it effectively blocks UVR at wavelengths less than 380 nm.

7.5.2.2 Use of interlocks. Interlocks are an essential requirement on source housings containing high-intensity UV lamps in order to prevent unnecessary and excessive exposure. However, if the housing contains a high-pressure arc lamp, such an interlock will not prevent the risk of injury from flying glass due to possible explosion of the lamp envelope, should the source housing be opened before the lamp has cooled down. Particular care should also be taken when high-pressure lamps are being removed or replaced; never handle a lamp by the quartz envelope since fingerprints or other contaminants can weaken the envelope.

7.5.2.3 Minimising reflected UVR. Many surfaces, such as polished metal, glass and high-gloss ceramic surfaces, are good reflectors of UVR. Reduction in reflected intensity can be achieved by coating the surface with a paint of low reflectance, although the ability of a material to reflect visible light is not necessarily a guide to its reflection in the UV. Table 7.5 lists the reflectance from a number of white pigments and other materials, and indicates that ordinary white wall plaster has a reflectance of 65% at 297 nm, whereas pressed zinc oxide and titanium oxide, which are equally good reflectors of visible light, reflect only 2.5% and 6% respectively at this wavelength. On the other hand, smoked magnesium oxide exhibits more than 90% reflectance throughout the UV and visible regions, and as such is sometimes used as the internal coating of integrating spheres designed for use in the ultraviolet.

Table 7.5 Reflectances of white pigments and other materials (Luckiesh 1946)

Material	Percent reflectance			
	254 nm	297 nm	365 nm	Visible light
Smoked magnesium oxide	93	93	94	95–97
White wall plaster	46	65	76	90
Titanium oxide	6	6	31	94
Pressed zinc oxide	2.5	2.5	4	88
Flat black Egyptian lacquer	5	5	5	5
Five samples of wallpaper	18–31	21–40	33–50	55–75

7.5.3 Personal protection

If adequate attention is given to administrative and engineering control measures, it may not be necessary to resort to personal protection, particularly skin protection. Nevertheless on some occasions the nature of the work in hand demands unavoidable exposure to UVR and in these instances appropriate personal protection should be taken. For example, a physicist may need to step inside a whole body UV irradiation unit to carry out irradiance measurements.

7.5.3.1 Skin protection. Protection of the skin against unnecessary exposure to UVR can be achieved by covering it with a material of suitable absorbing properties. Materials which transmit little UVR include poplin and flannelette, whereas white muslin batiste, cotton voile and nylon are relatively transparent. In general, tightly woven fabrics offer the best protection against actinic radiation, and colour and thickness are not necessarily a good guide to the suitability of protective clothing. Suitable gloves and face shields can be fabricated from polyvinyl chloride.

Where it proves impossible to shield the skin by suitable clothing, protection may still be achieved by sunscreens. Sunscreens are usually classified as chemical or physical. Chemical sunscreens act by absorbing the UVR and dissipating the energy as radiation of longer wavelength, and include such agents as para-aminobenzoic acid and its esters, cinnamates and salicylates. Physical agents, such as titanium dioxide and talcum powder, act by reflecting, absorbing or scattering the radiation.

To be an effective agent for blocking incident actinic radiation the sunscreen should possess the following qualities:

(a) high attenuation for radiation with wavelengths less than 315 nm;

(b) adherence to the skin under a variety of conditions, such as sweating, immersion of skin in water, and high and low humidity; and

(c) cosmetic acceptability.

7.5.3.2 Eye protection. Because of the sensitivity of the eye to UVR, it is good practice to wear adequate eye protection whenever there is the possibility of UV exposure. The principle acute ocular effect is kerato-conjunctivitis, which is initiated by radiation in the UV-C and UV-B regions. Chronic exposure to UV-A is thought to be a factor in producing cataracts. The council of perfection, therefore, is to wear glasses which are opaque to wavelengths less than 400 nm but that transmit an adequate amount of visible light so as not to be disorienting. Patients undergoing UV irradiation, particularly in physiotherapy departments, are usually given green tinted, occlusive goggles (for example, Portia, Actinotherapy Goggles, Solport Bros. Ltd.), whereas users of UV equipment may prefer to wear glasses which incorporate side-shields and combine negligible transmission in the UV spectrum with high transmission in the visible region (e.g. Blak-Ray Contrast Control Spectacles, Model No. UVC-303, Ultraviolet Products Inc.). Both these type of spectacle are illustrated in figure 7.8.

Patients who are taking photosensitising drugs as part of their treatment (e.g. PUVA patients) need to protect their eyes for as long as the drug is active. In the case of patients administered oral psoralens, this period needs to be the rest of the day, since solar UV-A irradiance can be as high as 50 W m^{-2}—a value which is comparable with that encountered in treatment units—and psoralons can be detected in human lenses for at least 12 h following oral ingestion (Lerman *et al* 1980).

In spite of the technical merits of glasses such as the Blak-Ray UVC-303 spectacles, and possibly other similar appliances, they cannot compete in cosmetic appeal with commercially available sun-spectacles incorporating tinted lenses. Some of these may in fact provide sufficient protection and, what is more important, the patient is likely actually to wear them.

Tinted lenses can be divided into two main groups. The first group comprises pure industrial filters which protect against harmful radiations on either side of the visible spectrum, both infrared and ultraviolet radiations and, in addition, reduce transmission within the visible spectrum. Sunglasses and tinted prescription lenses that have evolved from the original industrial glass materials are within this group. The second group are those where the principal consideration is the reduction of visible radiation, i.e. glare, and may or may not have protective properties as well. In addition, within this group are sunglasses which are worn principally for their cosmetic effect.

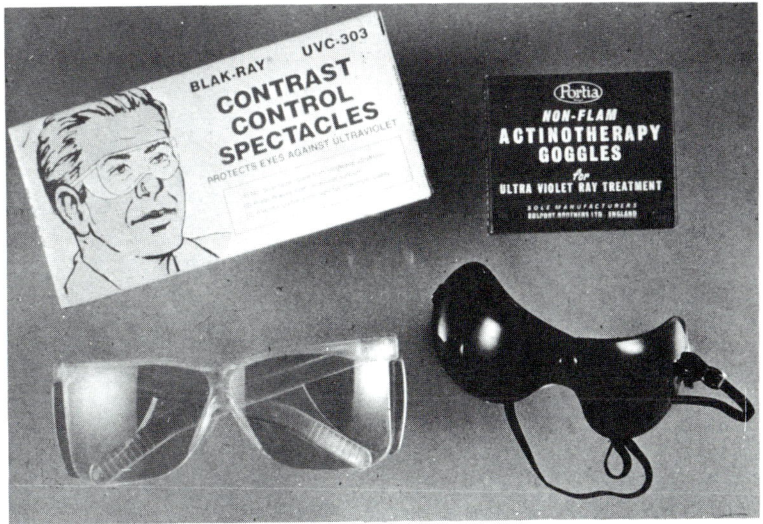

Figure 7.8 Two pairs of UV protective spectacles.

When protection against UV-A radiation is required, as in patients undergoing PUVA therapy, the first group, i.e. industrial filters and their derivatives, are unsuitable. Their function is to absorb well in the short UV (UV-B and UV-C) in order to prevent various forms of photo-ophthalmia. Although the denser shades of welding filters may provide protection agianst UV-A as well as the shorter UV wavelengths, they are so dark within the visible spectrum as to be impractical for non-industrial use. So industrial protective filters are unsuitable for patients who need protection against UV-A.

In general, non-polarising lenses have poorer properties of UVR absorption when compared with polarising lenses; indeed there are sunglasses available commercially which have a transmission of 30% or more at 300 nm.

Now that the hazard of the possible cataractogenic effects of UV-A on patients being treated with oral psoralen is appreciated it is possible that a lens which is opaque to wavelengths less than 400 nm but without a significant tint could be produced both in unpowered form for people who do not wear glasses for distance vision and also as a coating for those who require a powered lens to prescription. In the latter case it would seem a simple solution to use a plastics lens and then to treat its surface so as to give it the necessary absorption properties in the UV-A. This would eliminate the aversion response in which the pupil dilates in response to the decreased visible light levels associated with tinted lenses.

7.6 Hazards from Ozone

Ozone is a colourless, toxic, irritant gas and is formed from biatonic oxygen either by electric arc or corona discharges in air, or by a complex photochemical reaction between short-wavelength ultraviolet radiation and the oxygen present in the air. It is therefore possible to find ozone near ultraviolet lamps, especially those where radiation of wavelength shorter than about 250 nm is transmitted through the envelope of the lamp. There are many so-called 'ozone free' lamps available nowadays in which the lamp envelope is opaque to wavelengths below about 260 nm, thus preventing shorter-wavelength UVR from forming ozone in the air.

Ozone has a characteristic pungent odour which has been described as that of new-mown hay or sparking electrical machinery. It has been claimed by workers in the USSR that ozone can be detected by smell at a concentration as low as 0.005 ppm; other workers put the limit as high as 2 ppm. Detection by smell, therefore, may not provide adequate protection against occupational exposure. Olfactory fatigue occurs but one volunteer has clained that the ozone could still be smelt after 2 h of exposure to 1.5–2 ppm. The time-weighted average threshold limit value (TWA) for occupational exposure to ozone is currently given as 0.1 ppm by volume in air with the short-term (15 min) exposure limit tentatively set at 0.3 ppm (HSE 1978). This places ozone in the same toxicity class as carbonyl chloride (phosgene) (TWA = 0.1 ppm) and it is of higher toxicity than, for example, chlorine (TWA = 1 ppm) or carbon monoxide (TWA = 50 ppm). Exposure to ozone at a concentration of 50 ppm for 0.5 h may be fatal (EMAS 1972).

A simple, cheap and reliable way of estimating the concentration of ozone which may exist in the vicinity of an ultraviolet radiation emitting lamp is to use a Dräger tube (type ozone 0.05/a) and a Gastec pump. In this method a known volume of air is drawn through a glass tube packed with indigo. Ozone decomposes indigo into isatine, which is white, and the length of whitening corresponds to the ozone concentration. The glass tube is graduated in scale values of ppm ozone when 1000 ml of air (ten strokes of the piston) are drawn through the tube. Greater sensitivity can be achieved by increasing the number of strokes. The relative standard deviation of the estimate of concentration is about 10–15%. Ozone concentration is highest immediately after a UV lamp is struck, since, as the gas pressure rises, the short-wavelength UVR which produces ozone is reabsorbed more efficiently within the lamp.

If ozone is suspected, either by measurement or smell, steps should be taken to ensure adequate ventilation in the area around a source. One way is to connect the source housing to an exit port in an outside wall by means of ducting. A fan situated appropriately in the source housing should then serve to remove ozone, whilst cooling the lamp at the same time.

Further Reading

Blum H F 1959 *Carcinogenesis by Ultraviolet Light* (New Jersey: Princeton University)

Diffey B L (ed) 1978 *Ultraviolet Radiation and its Medical Applications* (Hospital Physicists' Association CRS-28)

Fitzpatrick T B (ed) 1974 *Sunlight and Man* (University of Tokyo)

Giese A C 1976 *Living with our Sun's Ultraviolet Rays* (New York: Plenum)

Harm W 1980 *Biological Effects of Ultraviolet Radiation* (Cambridge University)

Henderson S T 1970 *Daylight and its Spectrum* (New York: American Elsevier)

Henderson S T and Marsden A M (ed) 1972 *Lamps and Lighting* 2nd edn (London: Edward Arnold)

Hughes D 1978 *Hazards of Occupational Exposure to Ultraviolet Radiation* Occupational Hygiene Monograph No. 1 (University of Leeds Industrial Services)

Jagger J 1967 *Introduction to Research in Ultraviolet Photobiology* (New Jersey: Prentice-Hall)

Koller L R 1965 *Ultraviolet Radiation* 2nd edn (New York: John Wiley)

Licht S (ed) 1959 *Therapeutic Electricity and Ultraviolet Radiation* (Connecticut: Elizabeth Licht)

Magnus I A 1976 *Dermatological Photobiology* (Oxford: Blackwell)

Parrish J A, Anderson R R, Urbach F and Pitts D 1978 *UV-A: Biological Effects of Ultraviolet Radiation with Emphasis on Human Responses to Longwave Ultraviolet* (Chichester: John Wiley)

Regan J D and Parrish J A (ed) 1980 *The Science of Photomedicine* (New York: Plenum)

Sliney D and Wolbarsht M 1980 *Safety with Lasers and Other Optical Sources: A Comprehensive Handbook* (New York: Plenum)

Smith K C (ed) 1977 *The Science of Photobiology* (New York: Plenum)

Urbach F (ed) 1969 *The Biologic Effects of Ultraviolet Radiation with Emphasis on the Skin* (Oxford: Pergamon)

Wadsworth H and Chanmugam A P P 1980 *Electrophysical Agents in Physiotherapy* (Australia: Science Press)

References

ACGIH 1976 *Threshold Limit Values for Chemical Substances and Physical Agents in the Workroom Environment: Ultraviolet Radiation* (Cincinnati, Ohio: American Conference of Governmental Industrial Hygienists)

Bachem A 1956 *Am. J. Phys. Med.* **35** 177

Bachem A and Reed C I 1930 *Arch. Physical Therapy* **11** 49

Bener P 1972 *Final Technical Report DAJA37-68-C-1017* (London: European Research Office, U S Army)

Berger D, Urbach F and Davies R E 1968 In: *Proceedings 13th International Congress of Dermatology, Munich, 1967* (New York: Springer-Verlag) p 1112

Berger D S 1969 *J. Invest. Derm.* **53** 192

Boettner E A and Wolter J R 1962 *Invest. Ophthalmol.* **1** 776

Brodkin R H, Kopf A W and Andrade R 1969 In: *The Biologic Effects of Ultraviolet Radiation with Emphasis on the Skin* ed F Urbach (Oxford: Pergamon) p 581

Buck H W, Magnus I A and Porter A D 1960 *Br. J. Dermatol* **72** 249

Challoner A V J, Corless D, Davis A, Deane G H W, Diffey B L, Gupta S P and Magnus I A 1976 *Clin. Exp. Dermatol.* **1** 175

Claesson S, Juhlin L and Wettermark G 1958 *Acta Derm.-vener* **38** 123

Coblentz W W 1932 *Science* **76** 412

Commission Internationale de l'Eclairage 1970 *International Lighting Vocabulary* 3rd edn (Paris)

Corbett M F, Davis A and Magnus I A 1978 *Br. J. Dermatol.* **98** 39

Corless D, Gupta S P, Switala S, Barragry J M, Boucher B J, Cohen R D and Diffey B L 1978 *Lancet* September 23 649

Cremer R J, Peryman P W and Richards D H 1958 *Lancet* May 24 1094

Cripps D J and Ramsay C A 1970 *Br. J. Derm.* **82** 584

Cutler S J and Young J L 1975 *Natl. Cancer Inst. Monograph 41* (Washington D C: DHEW) **NIH** 75–707

Daniels F 1969 In: *The Biologic Effects of Ultraviolet Radiation with Emphasis on the Skin* ed F Urbach (Oxford: Pergamon) p 151

Davis A, Deane G H W and Diffey B L 1976 *Nature Lond.* **261** 169

Davis A, Diffey B L and Tate T J 1981 *Photochem. Photobiol.* **34** 283

Diffey B L 1977 *Phys. Med. Biol.* **22** 309

Diffey B L, Challoner A V J and Key P J 1980 *Br. J. Dermatol.* **102** 301

Diffey B L, Harrington T R and Challoner A V J 1978 *Br. J. Dermatol.* **99** 361

Diffey B L and Keir M I S 1977 *Proc. R. Soc. Med.* **70** 732

Diffey B L, Kerwin M and Davis A 1977 *Br. J. Dermatol.* **97** 407

Diffey B L, Larkö O and Swanbeck G 1982 *Br. J. Dermatol.* (in press)

Diffey B L and Mallion W E 1978 *Radiography* **44** 223

Diffey B L, Tate T J and Davis A 1979 *Phys. Med. Biol.* **24** 931

Dubertret L, Averbeck D, Zajdela F, Bisagni E, Moustacchi E, Touraine R and Latarjet R 1979 *Br. J. Dermatol.* **101** 379

EMAS 1972 *Ozone, Notes of Guidance* (London Chief Employment Medical Adviser, Health and Safety Executive)

Everett M A, Olson R L and Sayre R M 1965 *Arch. Dermatol.* **92** 713

Everett M A, Yeargers E, Sayre R M and Olson R L 1966 *Photochem. Photobiol.* **5** 533

Fears T R, Scotto J and Schneiderman M A 1977 *Am. J. Epidemiol.* **105** 420

Fischer T and Alsins J 1976 *Acta Dermatol.* **56** 383

Freeman R G, Owens D W, Knox J M and Hudson H T 1966 *J. Invest. Dermatol.* **47** 506

Freeman R G and Troll D 1969 *J. Invest. Dermatol.* **53** 449

Fry L 1977 *Br. J. Dermatol.* **96** 327

Gilchrest B A, Rowe J W, Brown R S, Steiman T I and Arndt K A 1977 *New Eng. J. Med.* **297** 136

Green A E S 1978 *Am. J. Epidemiol.* **107** 277

Green A E S, Cross K R and Smith L A 1980 *Photochem. Photobiol.* **31** 59

Green A E S, Findley G B, Klenk K F, Wilson W M and Mo T 1976 *Photochem. Photobiol.* **24** 353

Green A E S, Sawada T and Shettle E P 1974 *Photochem. Photobiol.* **19** 251

HSE 1978 *Threshold Limit Values for 1978, Guidance Note EH15* (London, HMSO: Health and Safety Executive)

Hanid M A and Levi A J 1980 *Lancet* September 6 530

Hansen K G 1948 *Acta Radiologica Suppl.* **71**

Hausser K W and Vahle W 1922 *Strahlentherapie* **13** 41

Henderson S T and Marsden A M 1972 *Lamps and Lighting* 2nd edn (London: Edward Arnold)

International Commission on Illumination, Berlin 1935 *Compt. Rend.* **9** 596

Johns H E and Rauth A M 1965 *Photochem. Photobiol.* **4** 673

Leach J F, McLeod V E, Pingstone A R, Davis A and Deane G H W 1978 *Clin. Exp. Dermatol.* **3** 77

Lerman S, Megaw J and Willis I 1980 *J. Invest Dermatol.* **74** 197

van der Leun J C 1966 *PhD. Thesis* (Univ. Utrecht, The Netherlands)

Luckiesh M 1946 *Applications of Germicidal, Erythermal and Infrared Energy* (New York: Van Nostrand) p 383

McCullough E C 1970 *Phys. Med. Biol* **15** 723

Mackenzie L A and Frain-Bell W 1973 *Br. J. Dermatol.* **89** 251

Magnus I A 1976 *Dermatological Photobiology* (Oxford: Blackwell)

Magnus I A, Porter A D, McCree K J, Moreland J D and Wright W D 1959 *Br. J. Dermatol.* **71** 261

Mathews-Roth M M, Pathak M A, Fitzpatrick T B, Harber L C and Kass E H 1974 *J. Am. Med. Assoc.* **228** 1004

Melles Griot 1975 *Optics Guide* (Arnhem, Holland: Melles Griot)

Nakayama Y, Morikawa F, Fukuda M, Hamano M R, Toda K and Pathak M A 1974 In: *Sunlight and Man* ed Fitzpatrick T B (University of Tokyo) p 591

National Institute for Occupational Safety and Health 1972 *Criteria for a Recommended Standard . . . Occupational Exposure to Ultraviolet Radiation* (Washington D C: DHEW)

National Radiological Protection Board 1977 *Protection against Ultraviolet Radiation in the Workplace* (London: HMSO) **ISBN** 0 85951 063 8

Owens D W, Glicksman J M, Freeman R G and Carnes R 1968 *J. Invest. Dermatol.* **51** 435

Palmer E W, Hutley M C, Franks A, Verrill J F and Gale B 1975 4 *Rep. Progr. Phys.* **38** 975

Parrish J A, Anderson R R, Urbach F and Pitts D 1978 *UV-A: Biological Effects of Ultraviolet Radiation with Emphasis on Human Responses to Longwave Ultraviolet* (Chichester: John Wiley)

Parrish J A, Fitzpatrick T B, Tanenbaum L and Pathak M A 1974 *New Eng. J. Med.* **291** 1207

Pathak M A 1961 *J. Invest. Dermatol.* **37** 397

Pitts D G 1973 *Health Physics* **25** 559

Saleeby C W 1926 *Sunlight and Health* 3rd edn (London: Nisbet) p 72

Schott 1970 *Color Filter Glass.* (Mainz, West Germany: Jenaer Glaswerk Schott)

Setlow R B 1974 *Proc. Nat. Acad. Sci. USA* **71** 3363

Stobbart D and Diffey B L 1980 *Clin. Phys. Physiol. Meas.* **1** 267

Urbach F, Epstein J H and Forbes P D 1974 In: *Sunlight and Man* ed Fitzpatrick T B (University of Tokyo) p 259

WHO 1979 *Environmental Health Criteria 14: Ultraviolet Radiation* (Geneva: WHO)

Index